Outpatient, Day Surgery and Ambulatory Care

Edited by

Lioba Howatson-Jones
PGCLT (HE), MHSCC (postgrad), Cert Ed, BSc (Hons), DipHE, RGN, ENB R26
Fellow of the Higher Education Academy
Senior Lecturer in Nursing and Applied Clinical Studies
Canterbury Christ Church University

and

Peter Ellis
MA, MSc, BSc (Hons), RN PGDip (LSH&TM), PGCE, PGCM, PGcert (Crit Care), ENB136
Senior Lecturer in Nursing and Applied Clinical Studies
Canterbury Christ Church University

WILEY-BLACKWELL
A John Wiley & Sons, Ltd., Publication

This edition first published 2008
© 2008 John Wiley & Sons, Ltd

Wiley-Blackwell is an imprint of John Wiley and Sons, formed by the merger of Wiley's global Scientific, Technical and Medical business with Blackwell Publishing

Registered office
John Wiley & Sons Ltd, The Atrium, Southern Gate, Chichester, West Sussex, PO19 8SQ, United Kingdom

Editorial office
John Wiley & Sons Ltd, The Atrium, Southern Gate, Chichester, West Sussex, PO19 8SQ, United Kingdom

For details of our global editorial offices, for customer services and for information about how to apply for permission to reuse the copyright material in this book please see our website at www.wiley.com/wiley-blackwell.

A catalogue record for this book is available from the British Library.

Library of Congress Cataloging-in-Publication Data

Outpatient, day surgery, and ambulatory care / edited by Lioba Howatson-Jones and Peter Ellis.
     p.   ; cm.
   Includes bibliographical references and index.
   ISBN 978-0-470-51283-8 (pbk. : alk. paper)   1. Ambulatory surgical nursing–Great Britain.
2. Primary care (Medicine)–Great Britain.   I. Howatson-Jones, Lioba. II. Ellis, Peter, 1969-
   [DNLM: 1. Ambulatory Care–trends–Great Britain.   2. Nurse's Role–Great Britain.   3. Ambulatory Surgical Procedures–nursing–Great Britain.   4. Health Knowledge, Attitudes, Practice–Great Britain.
5. Primary Health Care–trends–Great Britain. WY 150   094   2008]
   RD110.5.098 2008
   617′.0231–dc22

                                                                                         2008006731

Set in 10/12 pt Sabon by Aptara Inc., New Delhi, India
Printed in Singapore by Markono Print Media Pte Ltd

1   2008

Contents

Contributors

Peter Ellis, MA, MSc, BSc(Hons), RN PGDip (LSH&TM), PGCE, PGCM, PGcert (Crit Care), ENB136, is a Senior Lecturer in Nursing and Applied Clinical Studies at Canterbury Christ Church University. Peter's areas of interest are research, renal nursing, management and ethics. Prior to joining Christ Church Peter was a Senior Nurse for Renal Outpatients and Research Projects Manager at King's College Hospital London and has tutored the renal course at Kingston University and King's College London.

Roger Goldsmith, MSc, BA, RGN, RNT, is a Senior Lecturer in Nursing and Applied Clinical Studies at Canterbury Christ Church University. Roger's areas of interest are advanced nursing practice, academic development and emergency care. Prior to joining Canterbury Christ Church, Roger was a clinical teacher in Accident and Emergency at Medway Maritime Hospital. He also works part-time as an Emergency Nurse Practitioner at the nurse-led minor injury unit at Kent and Canterbury Hospital, East Kent Hospitals NHS Trust.

Lioba Howatson-Jones, PGCLT (HE), MHSCC (post-grad), Cert Ed, BSc (Hons), DipHE, RGN, ENB R26, is a Fellow of the Higher Education Academy and Senior Lecturer in Nursing and Applied Clinical Studies at Canterbury Christ Church University. She leads on the pre-registration module for outpatient and day service care. Lioba's areas of interest are research, radiological services, women's health, nurse education and academic development. Prior to joining Canterbury Christ Church Lioba was a Practice Development Nurse and Radiology Nurse in East Kent Hospitals NHS Trust.

Paula Kuzbit, MSc, PGCLT, BSc(Hons), DipN, RN, ENB 237, is the Professional Lead for Adult Nursing and a Senior Lecturer in Nursing and Applied Clinical Studies at Canterbury Christ Church University. Paula's areas of interest are cancer care, nursing education, practice development and the patient's experience. Before joining Canterbury Christ Church University Paula was the Oncology Practice Development Nurse at the Kent Oncology Centre.

Karen Lumsden, BSc(Hons)Nurse Practitioner, RGN, ENB 199, A33, is a Senior Lecturer Practitioner in Nursing and Applied Clinical Studies at Canterbury Christchurch University. Karen's areas of interest are emergency and critical care, major incident planning and trauma care. As a Senior Sister she divides her time equally between academia and clinical practice working within A&E services.

Beverley McNeil, PGCLT(HE), MSc, LPE, BSc(Hons), ENB 183, RGN, is a Fellow of the Higher Education Academy and a Senior Lecturer in Nursing and Applied Clinical Studies at Canterbury Christ Church University. Beverley has a particular interest in surgery, operating theatre practice, CJD and decontamination and currently lectures on the operating department practitioner and adult nursing programmes. Prior to joining the university staff, Beverley was a Theatre Sister with East Kent Hospitals NHS Trust.

Des Nolan, MSc, DipNEd, RNT, RCNT, RGN, ENB 934, is a Senior Lecturer in Nursing and Applied Clinical Studies at Canterbury Christ Church University. Des's areas of interest include palliative care, bereavement and spirituality.

Judith Parsons, MSc, BA, PGCEA, PG Dip, RN, DN, NP, RNT, is a Senior Lecturer in the Department of Social Work, Community and Mental Health at Canterbury Christ Church University. Judith Parsons has worked as a district nurse and has been involved in community nursing education for a number of years. She currently leads a masters route for community matrons and is interested in new roles in community nursing. She also contributes to community nursing modules in pre-registration nursing programmes.

Sarah Pye, MA, BSc(Hons), District Nurse, RGN, is a Senior Lecturer who is currently the programme director for Independent and Supplementary prescribing for Nurses and Midwives and supplementary prescribing for allied health professionals. She is currently the module leader for a primary care module for the adult nursing pathway. Sarah has worked as a district nurse for 7 years. Before moving into education Sarah has worked on many projects in primary care including the introduction of NHS continuing care. Sarah is interested in the development of non-medical prescribing, advanced nursing practice and leadership development for nurses.

Colin Wheeldon, postgraduate certificate in Interprofessional Health and Community Care, BA(Hons), Dip. Cont Ed, Cert Ed. RGN, ENB 978, is a Senior Lecturer in Nursing and Applied Clinical Studies at Canterbury Christ Church University. Colin's areas of interest are moving and handling (patients), the student experience of higher education, pre-registration recruitment and retention, promotion of continence and management of incontinence.

Preface

The purpose of the book

Day services and outpatient settings cover a broad spectrum of practice areas in acute hospitals interfacing with primary care. This is a rapidly expanding field and at the forefront of the government agenda. The principle aim of this book is to provide a text that encompasses central areas of ambulatory care provision and develop a critical awareness of the evidence base for decision making in short-term practice arenas. The book covers a wide range of diagnostic and short-stay therapeutic provision including minor injuries, day surgery, outpatients, radiology, endoscopy, renal care, oncology ambulatory clinics, day hospitals and the links with primary care. It focuses on specific nursing issues and the developing role of the nurse within each of these areas of practice. The book explores the broad knowledge base required of nurses working in these arenas, as well as the ability to communicate effectively within the multidisciplinary team. It brings together the relationships between areas through scenarios to give a more integrated view of short-term care settings and to reflect the patient journey in one text. This enables the reader to review, reflect on and enhance their own knowledge base. This process is referred to throughout the book as cumulative knowledge.

The book is written primarily for experienced student nurses who have moved beyond the common foundation programme of their preparation course and who are extending their scope of practice and level of nursing care decision making in adult settings. It will also be relevant to newly qualified nurses entering a short-term care arena, as well as experienced practitioners moving from other areas of care or those wishing to acquaint themselves with specific patient preparation and aftercare.

The development process of the book

The book developed from an innovative module in the pre-registration curriculum that introduced student nurses, in their second year, to caring for patients in outpatient and day service settings. The authors recognised the shift to more ambulatory services and an increasing focus on primary care provision. Existing texts were dated and none assimilated principle ambulatory settings into one book. Students also expressed difficulty in locating relevant literature.

Review of the book proposal by other institutions indicated a real need for such a text as many of the settings given priority here appeared only as addendums in other books. Coverage of developments within primary care and policy were viewed as particularly relevant. The integrated scenarios were thought to be especially helpful in enabling students to build on their knowledge of the nature of the patient journey. Opportunities for student reflection in practice were highly regarded. Review of the chapters by practice colleagues have also indicated interest in such a text from the areas that it covers. A practical approach was used to develop the book to appeal to undergraduate students in the main, but also to offer a source of reference to more experienced practitioners requiring specific information. The book focus is based on relevant procedures and current and future developments of the nursing role.

Organisation of the book

The chapters are organised to reflect the patient journey. An overarching chapter on communication and advocacy applied to the short-term setting begins the book. Developments in primary care provide threads which are referred to in all the subsequent chapters. The journey approach features the likely initial contact with services through outpatient and minor injury/illness settings, through pre-assessment and diagnostic environments, to day surgery and ambulatory settings such as renal and oncology and finishing with rehabilitative care in day hospitals. This approach suggests to the reader the likely experiences patients may have undergone before arriving in their particular setting, and what to look for in documentation. It also offers a holistic view of that experience.

Features

'Cumulative knowledge', 'checkpoint', 'reflection' and 'opportunity for the student' boxes appear within the text to raise critical questions and enable the reader to assimilate information between chapters. Scenarios that follow the patient journey between settings and chapters offer worked examples for the reader to engage with. These have been used and tested within the pre-registration module generating critical decision making. Images of specialist equipment are used, where relevant, such as the theatre environment and to enhance explanation. Specialist websites are offered at the end of each chapter to direct the reader to further sources of information. A glossary of specialist terms used in the chapter is also offered to enhance understanding.

Acknowledgements

The editors acknowledge the help of the following people in sharing ideas and helping to develop the project. Those involved in the development of specific chapters are acknowledged at the end of that section.

Fiona McCarthur-Rouse for helpful advice on putting a project together and tips of pitfalls to be avoided.
Carrie Sanders, head of department, for supporting the project.
Peers and practice colleagues who contributed to discussions on relevant topics.
The anonymous reviewers for their helpful feedback on draft manuscripts of the book.
The helpful publishing staff for their advice and guidance.
Our families for their support during the writing and editing of this book.

Chapter 1

Introduction

Lioba Howatson-Jones and Peter Ellis

The policy context

Current UK government policy is committed to shifting health care provision from the secondary care sector (the acute hospital) to the primary care sector (the community). New services, particularly those expanding into primary care, enable patients to access and receive attention more conveniently than would be the case if they had to travel to hospital (Department of Health (DH), 2007a). The consultation undertaken as part of 'Our health, Our care, Our say' (DH, 2006a) identifies that patients, their families and carers prefer to be treated closer to home – advances in surgery have made this possible by enabling routine surgery to be undertaken outside of the acute hospital setting.

The move from outpatient provision in the acute to community care settings is also prevalent within other health care systems such as that in the United States of America where in 1981 90% of appointments were in the hospital, but by 2003 this had reduced to 50% (DH, 2006a, p. 32).

The National Health Service plan and National Service Frameworks for specific health care priorities aim to reduce the dependence on inpatient care by investing in community-based services (DH, 2007b). The reconfiguration of health care services is aimed at expanding the services provided by general practitioners, nurses, midwives and pharmacists whilst enabling them to develop specialist skills making it possible for them to take on new responsibilities, such as follow-up treatments, testing, post-surgical checks and some minor operative procedures (DH, 2007c).

The increased provision of diagnostic as well as treatment services is aimed at enabling faster access to health care (DH, 2005). The UK government has set an 18-week limit on the patient pathway from time of referral to start of treatment. This target includes outpatient, diagnostic investigations as well as inpatient stages of the patient journey (DH, 2006b). The focus is on a patient-driven, locally focused health service delivering a quality patient experience (DH, 2006c). Patients are to be given greater choice in their health care as outpatient and day services are located in a broader spectrum of practice arenas in both acute hospitals and primary care.

Aims and objectives of the book

The principle aim of this book is to help the novice, or new, practitioner to develop an appreciation of the diversity, and potential, for the provision of care in the outpatient setting as well as cultivate a critical awareness evidence base for decision making in short-term practice arenas. This text considers provision of care in ambulatory settings and assimilates key areas, including developing services in primary care, minor injuries, day surgery, outpatients, radiology, endoscopy, renal clinics, oncology ambulatory clinics and day hospitals, into one text.

Recent technological advancements in lighting, digital imaging, instrumentation and pharmacology have made it possible for many procedures that traditionally required an overnight admission to hospital to now be carried out on a day-case, ambulatory basis. Short-acting anaesthetics and conscious sedation make it possible for patients to undergo invasive procedures with a quick recovery time. These advances generate a fast pace of work, which requires that practitioners are able to function autonomously and where patients increasingly participate in their own care. Patients may move between being independent and dependent very rapidly and may exhibit complications suddenly. Good communication and assessment skills are a vital part of working in this environment and it is intended that the reader will be able to use the opportunities highlighted in the individual chapters to develop these skills in relation to the given subject.

Structure of the book

The development of day services places considerable demands on health care professionals as they seek to establish a therapeutic relationship with their patients during a shorter period of interaction. Acquiring and using appropriate interpersonal skills helps practitioners to understand and respond more adequately to their patients' needs and concerns and to plan individualised care. By helping patients to make decisions for themselves, they are able to gain a sense of ownership for their own health care needs and are more likely to participate in health promotion activities. Practitioners, at times, may need to adopt the role of patient advocate by supporting patients who have difficulty in being able to make decisions for themselves or who are unable to do so for one reason or another. The role of the outpatient practitioner/student is, therefore, one which involves good communication. Establishing a therapeutic relationship is fundamental to good patient care, and key to being able to establish this relationship is the exercise of first-class interpersonal skills.

Chapter 2 provides an overarching view of communication and advocacy and how these concepts relate to working in short-term settings. It offers insight into patients' experiences of day services and introduces themes and ideas, which are developed further in the individual chapters, to help practitioners to recognise and respond to their patients' needs in this time-limited setting. Examples of interpersonal skills are given and a brief explanation of their use examined. Empowering patients to make informed decisions and choices about health care interventions is also explored.

Developments in primary care are reducing the demand for hospital-based services. Patients no longer have to travel to the acute hospital for operations that can be performed as a day case. Outpatient services are increasingly available in the community setting. Patients requiring rehabilitation and management of exacerbations of long-term conditions can also receive hospital-type care in their own homes. Cancer patients in some areas receive chemotherapy in the community. All these services are reducing the demand for beds and services in acute hospital settings. Chapter 3 explores developments in health care and how they have increased the range of services available to patients in their own homes or in alternative settings. It considers the importance of inter-agency and inter-professional collaboration in facilitating an efficient patient journey through this evolving health care system. The role of nurses in the development of primary care services is discussed in relation to day and outpatient services. The potential risk associated with the transfer of care from acute to primary care is also considered.

Outpatient clinics cater to a wide range of conditions, specialties and patient populations and are often the first contact that patients have with a specialist service. Nursing in an outpatient setting, whether in the community or in a hospital department, requires a comprehensive knowledge base and the ability to engage with patients in a short space of time whilst facilitating them in making informed choices.

Chapter 4 covers two main areas exploring the function and activity of the outpatient service and discussing the partnership established between the patient and the nurse in making choices about care decisions. Patient expectations and concerns about equality, organisation, efficiency and accurate information are related to personal values which may also impact on the nature and value of health promotion activities within the outpatients setting.

Minor injury and minor illness management is a dynamic and significant part of emergency and primary care in the UK. The course of a minor problem is usually short, although some can relapse. Symptoms are such that the patient can be discharged home with appropriate resources. Caring for patients in this setting means the nurse will need to be familiar with a wide variety of injury and illness pathologies among individuals from across the lifespan, differing social classes, different ethnicities, economic backgrounds and community settings. Chapter 5 explores different assessment models and specific strategies employed by nurses in the context of a multidisciplinary team requiring effective communication and management skills. Opportunities for the student are highlighted with regard to individualised person-centred care and reflection on ethical principles and informed consent.

Political pressure to reduce waiting times for procedures and cancellations has highlighted aspects of the patient experience which could be improved. One area is in ensuring that patients are adequately prepared for their examination and conversant with what to expect. A number of patients experience great uncertainty and apprehension regarding forthcoming events, and improved information giving and alleviation of that uncertainty and apprehension may result in lower 'no show' rates. The main objective of preoperative assessment in a surgical setting is to ensure fitness of the patient for surgery and anaesthesia within a day surgery unit and to ensure a complete understanding of the proposed surgery. Chapter 6 provides an overview of the pre-assessment process, including the need for reassessment, and the importance of effective pre-assessment in reducing patient cancellations. It explains the criteria used to assess fitness for surgery in a day care setting and considers the role of the pre-assessment practitioner in terms of autonomous working and communicating across teams and service boundaries. Opportunities for the student and novice practitioner in terms of communication, health promotion and pharmacological knowledge are also identified.

Radiological nursing requires a large knowledge base regarding a wide range of procedures. The nursing role is embedded within the multidisciplinary team in an arena which is very public. The team membership, ephemeral nature of the nurse–patient relationship and the very public nature of the radiology department mean that this is an area in which nurses require good advocacy skills. Chapter 7 considers this area of nursing practice and is divided into two sections. In part one, issues related to radiology as a specialty are considered with the science of imaging modalities explained and discussion in physiological terms including some of the various types of contrast used for enhancing imaging. Health and safety are also considered with regard to radiation risk, infection control and manual handling. The role of the nurse in creating an atmosphere of trust, providing assistance and future role developments, is also examined. In part two, general diagnostic and interventional procedures are considered with respect to care requirement and nursing input. Opportunities for the student in relation to broadening their knowledge about health and safety are offered.

As technology has developed, a greater variety of patients and conditions have presented for diagnostic and therapeutic intervention. Endoscopy nursing has followed developments in this field of practice, with nurses increasingly taking on roles previously carried out by other professionals. Chapter 8 considers issues in the science of endoscopic visualisation and explores developing modalities. Health and safety are related to care of endoscopic equipment and decontamination as part of infection control. The nursing role is explored in relation to care aspects and management strategies of selected procedures undertaken in the endoscopy environment. The developing role of the nurse endoscopist and future progression are also considered. Opportunities for the student are highlighted.

Patients undergoing a surgical procedure will require local, general or regional anaesthesia or, for some procedures, conscious sedation. The patient's pathway through day surgery covers admission on the day of surgery, the various ways in which anaesthesia/analgesia may be administered, intra-operative care, recovery and postoperative considerations followed by the criteria which must be met prior to the patient's safe discharge from the day surgery unit. Nurses working within the operating theatre have a clear understanding of their role within the day surgery unit and the importance of adhering to local and national guidelines and principles, which make for the smooth running of the unit. In Chapter 9, a brief overview of the patient's perioperative journey is outlined, from admission, through surgery, to discharge. The chapter gives the reader a broad overview of the work undertaken by the multidisciplinary team within a day surgery unit, through documenting the care requirements of patients systematically progressing through their perioperative journey. The reader will gain some insight into life behind the scenes of the day surgery ward and theatre environment.

Opportunities for role development for both nurses and operating department practitioners are currently at an exciting stage. The student is, therefore, encouraged to be proactive in seeking opportunities to follow patients through their surgical episode in order that this challenging and rewarding environment can be experienced.

Working in renal care offers a wide variety of opportunities. The care of the renal patient ranges from community-based screening and management of early renal disease through inpatient care, chronic and acute dialysis and ultimately palliative and terminal care. This variety means that the renal practitioner is presented with a myriad of choices as to where to practice and exercise both their chronic and acute skills. Chapter 10 identifies the physiological functions of the kidneys and the causes, classifications and effects of renal disease and discusses some of the many outpatient settings in which renal care is provided whilst also highlighting the important role that inter-professional working has in attaining a high quality of care. This chapter goes some way towards demonstrating that renal outpatient areas provide a diverse, challenging and engaging place for the health student to gain a unique insight into true inter-professional, patient-centred care.

Cancer care occurs in a wide variety of settings, including inpatient facilities, primary care and the ambulatory care setting. A considerable issue facing today's cancer services is the number of treatment episodes patients are experiencing. Current services are struggling to meet this increased demand, and new ways of working and delivering care are essential. The nurse's role is fundamental in supporting patients by providing in-depth information and education, ensuring the safety of the patient whilst they are at home and giving high levels of psychosocial and physical support. In Chapter 11, ambulatory cancer care and the role of the nurse are discussed, including current and potential developments. The purpose of chemotherapy, radiotherapy and biotherapy in the treatment of cancer is described with implications for nursing practice highlighted. Supportive care offered to cancer patients in the day care setting is also examined. Opportunities for the student in terms of identifying potential side effects and advisory information are offered.

The day hospital supports patients that need up to 8 hours of care in the day. It provides clinical consultation, diagnostic function tests and defined and time-limited multidisciplinary rehabilitation care packages of 6–12 weeks predominantly for older people. Chapter 12 defines the role of the day hospital and discusses the context of care, client groups and current developments in moving to medical ambulatory care. The role of the nurse within the interdisciplinary team is examined in terms of opportunities and future developments. Health promotion activities are identified and form part of the opportunity for the student to further develop their nursing skills.

The concluding chapter draws the main threads of ambulatory care together and considers what next. It draws on a view of the critically active practitioner who applies known principles in this short-term setting and recognises new effects and future actions. Fundamental to critical practice is maintaining a questioning approach to the provision of care and continuing to develop one's understanding, not only of the disease processes which affect people but also of their psychological and social responses to ill health. Health care provision is recognised as being complex and multifaceted and requiring that the student and developing practitioner understand their own role, the role of other professions and the role of the patient in providing safe care which is both effective and acceptable to the patient.

This book seeks to provide the reader with opportunities to explore the interaction between policy, procedure, evidence, physical, psychological and truly interdisciplinary working. It is suggested that the student takes the opportunities highlighted within the text and seeks to explore them by means of reading other textbooks and articles where appropriate. It is also suggested that the student uses the text to frame questions to discuss with their tutors, mentors and other professional colleagues as they explore practice within this growth area.

Most importantly, the student is encouraged to reflect on their own practice, the practice of others and the experience of health care provision. Reflection exposes thoughts, feelings and assumptions about situations that are often obscured in the day-to-day business of practice. By analysing these aspects and the knowledge in use, the student is able to develop critical questions and look for potential solutions that build new ways of working. Such reflection may be undertaken alone, with others students and other professionals. Guided reflection in the form of clinical supervision is particularly helpful for the novice practitioner to make sense of new situations and their own responses and to develop reflective ability in a safe/supportive environment. Discussion with and understanding of the patients' experiences of care are necessary in attaining some insight into how to best provide care in the various outpatient settings within which the student will find themselves working.

Acknowledgement

The editors thank Richard Hayward, senior lecturer, Canterbury Christ Church University, for his advice on policy and for helping in reading the manuscript.

References

Department of Health (DH) (2005) Press release. *Speedier Scans for Patients as Choice Rolls out to Diagnostics* [online]. Available from: http://www.dh.gov.uk/en/Publicationsandstatistics/Pressreleases/DH_4116422 (accessed 12 January 2007).

Department of Health (DH) (2006a) *The White Paper Command Paper: Our Health, Our Care, Our Say* [online]. Available from: http://www.dh.gov.uk/en/Publicationsandstatistics/Publications/PublicationsPolicyAndGuidance/DH_4127453 (accessed 12 October 2007).

Department of Health (DH) (2006b) *Working Towards the 18 Week Patient Pathway* [online]. Available from: http://www.dh.gov.uk/en/News/DH_4134616 (accessed 12 October 2007).

Department of Health (DH) (2006c) *Health Reform in England: Update and Commissioning Framework* [online]. Available from: http://www.dh.gov.uk/en/Publicationsandstatistics/Publications/PublicationsPolicyAndGuidance/DH_4137226 (accessed 12 October 2007).

Department of Health (DH) (6 September 2007a) News 6/09/2007. *Our NHS, Our Future: NHS Next Stage Review – Interim Report* [online]. Available from: http://www.dh.gov.uk/en/News/DH_078296 (accessed 12 October 2007).

Department of Health (DH) (2007b) *Breaking Down Barriers: The Clinical Case for Change. Report Professor Louis Appleby, National Director Mental Health* [online]. Available from: http://www.dh.gov.uk/en/Publicationsandstatistics/Publications/PublicationsPolicyAndGuidance/DH_074579 (accessed 12 October 2007).

Department of Health (DH) (2007c) *Keeping It Personal. Clinical Case for Change: Report by David Colin-Thome, National Director for Primary Care* [online]. Available from: http://www.dh.gov.uk/en/Publicationsandstatistics/Publications/PublicationsPolicyAndGuidance/DH_065094 (accessed 12 October 2007).

Chapter 2

Communication and advocacy

Des Nolan and Peter Ellis

Learning objectives

(1) Explore communication strategies and effective interpersonal skills when providing care for patients in day care settings
(2) Discuss the concept of empowerment and the role of the nurse in helping patients make informed decisions
(3) Examine the role of the nurse as an advocate for patients

Introduction

Definition

The establishment of a therapeutic relationship between nurses and their patients is essential in any care setting. Whilst in many areas this relationship appears to develop with relative ease, the short stay associated with day settings would appear to mitigate against this (Rogan and Timmins, 2004). This chapter discusses some of the strategies which may be applied in the outpatient setting when attempting to create a rapport with patients who are seen only for short periods of time. This chapter also discusses and defines the role of the nurse in empowering and advocating for patients in this setting.

The provision of day services and outpatient settings is a rapidly expanding field of health care and is central to the government agenda. New technologies, financial pressures and changes within society generally appear to be driving these changes. Improving the experience of the individual accessing health care and day services is central to this programme (Department of Health, 2000).

Initial consultation on the National Health Service plan demonstrated that patients wanted help when using heath services as these often appeared intimidating for them, and more so if things went wrong. Patients also voiced their concerns about the need to be more involved in making decisions about their own health care needs (Otte, 1996). From the practitioner's point of view, there are clearly issues around empowering patients to make necessary decisions which will ultimately also impact them.

Much has been written about the patient–practitioner relationship (Arnold and Undermann Boggs, 2003; Sully and Dallas, 2005). The quality of the care provided and the importance of establishing a relationship of trust between the practitioner and the patient would seem to be key to this process. Central to establishing a rapport is the need for effective communication; this requires that the practitioner develops the necessary interpersonal skills in order to be able to respond more effectively to their patients' needs. The establishment of successful relationships between practitioners and patients may be easier within inpatient settings where the patient stay is longer (for example medical and surgical wards), but more difficult in short-stay settings where patients are only in for a few hours or a day (Rogan and Timmins, 2004).

This chapter provides an overview of issues related to communicating with patients attending for short-stay investigations and interventions. It introduces ideas about communication and advocacy that are developed further in relation to specific settings in the subsequent chapters. The chapter begins by providing some background information relating to the development of day services and the rationale for expansion of such services. It offers some insight into patients' experiences of using such services. This in turn determines the way in which themes and ideas are developed in relation to helping practitioners to more ably recognise and respond to their patients' needs. The importance of establishing a therapeutic relationship is explored, focusing in particular on the acquisition and development of interpersonal skills. Examples of these skills are offered and a brief explanation of their use is examined.

The second half of the chapter explores issues associated with empowering patients to make informed decisions and choices about health care interventions. It also discusses how to support patients who, for one reason or another, may need the practitioner to act as an advocate on their behalf. Whilst for many patients the experience of being an inpatient on a day surgical unit may go smoothly, for others the experience may be less satisfactory.

Developing a therapeutic relationship

The establishment of any relationship begins the moment the practitioner meets the patient entrusted to their care. The initial greeting is important, as this may be the first time that the patient engages with an investigation or intervention. Alternatively, it may be the patient's second or third attendance and they might be worrying about being 'called back' again for further tests and fearing the worst, particularly if the first admission and intervention had failed to ameliorate a health problem.

Upon arrival, the patient is greeted and made to feel welcome. A handshake is a customary way of greeting another person and demonstrates that the practitioner is welcoming and beginning to want to engage with their patient. It may be useful to establish how the patient likes to be addressed and whether they do indeed use the name as it appears on their notes.

The practitioner provides a brief overview of the plan of care for the patient and any associated interventions. It is in these early stages that the practitioner ascertains how the patient may be feeling, their level of understanding about any intervention and any questions they may have about any aspect of their care. Strategies which allow the practitioner to ascertain whether the individual has understood what is being discussed include the use of general questions that range from 'do you understand what I mean by ...' to providing permission for the patient to question what has been said: 'have you got any questions about what I just said'. Where doubt exists as to the level of understanding, simple prompts like 'can you tell me what you understand about the procedure' may help the nurse to identify what the patient has in fact understood.

Whether it is the patient's first encounter with day services or not, the prospect of meeting a health care professional and undergoing tests and procedures can seem quite daunting. Patients are likely to have numerous concerns and questions about the reason for their attendance, and gentle questioning allows opportunity for the patient to voice these concerns.

Concerns which may not be immediately obvious to the practitioner may relate to whether the patient feels that they will be able to go back to work the following day or relate to care responsibilities, such as childcare, while they are away. Understanding and empathising about the human elements of caring goes a long way towards helping to develop a rapport with patients.

Other anxieties include not understanding medical terminology and jargon that health care professionals might use in relation to the procedure itself, findings during or after the intervention, and follow-up care. These are easily addressed by establishing the patient's level of understanding through gentle questioning and then tailoring the language used to match their ability to understand. Even health care professionals receiving care for a condition which is not within their area of expertise appreciate a lay explanation!

There may also be concerns around being given bad news, for example an unfavourable diagnosis. Any unexpected news for the patient about their health is likely to create anxiety for them, with fears relating to how they will respond when it is given and later on, and how they might feel when they have had time to reflect on it. All these issues clearly have implications for those who are caring for them (Smeltzer and Bare, 2004). The impact of such events is reduced if the patient has a good rapport with their nurse and if they feel that they can express their fears and worries and will receive both time and support.

It would appear then that the key figure in terms of supporting the patient at this time is the nurse who has been assigned to care for the patient during their stay and with whom a positive rapport needs to be developed. This association is often referred to as a therapeutic relationship. Establishing any effective relationship requires the practitioner to show a genuine interest in their patient and demonstrate a degree of acceptance of them and empathy towards them during their journey (Stein-Parbury, 2000).

Imparting the health care message may mean that the nurse has to repeat the health care message or interpret some aspect of communication that was given to the patient earlier which they may not have understood. For example the surgeon may have given the patient a diagnosis following an investigation, but it is very often the nurse who may find them self-explaining what was meant by certain words and phrases used during an earlier conversation. Patients need to be supported when being given such information in order to help them make a decision about a medical intervention, and this may include family members or significant others. In this way the nurse is beginning to collate information so that a plan of care can be compiled for that patient during their stay, and engage in pre-assessment as discussed more fully in Chapter 6.

Consideration also needs to be given to the barriers of effective communication. Some procedures may be viewed as highly embarrassing for patients, for example a cystoscopy performed whilst the patient is awake, or having to pass urine whilst an X-ray is taken. Paying attention to the environment in which the communication takes place and ensuring that there is some privacy and that the patient can feel at ease is an important step in overcoming barriers to communication. The protection of privacy and dignity is a fundamental part of the role of the nurse and is a requirement of good quality care (National Health Service Modernisation Agency, 2003). Further skills may be required when communicating with people with physical or mental impairment or learning difficulties. These skills are outside the scope of this text and readers should refer to more specialist texts for help in these areas.

In order to examine these skills and put them into some kind of context, it might be helpful to reflect on the findings from some of the research which sought the views of users/patients accessing day care settings. The findings clearly have important things to say in relation to improving the relationship between practitioner and patient, and the important part that communication plays in helping to foster and develop this relationship.

> **Reflection**
>
> What potential barriers to effective communication might present themselves in the above-mentioned procedures?

Developing interpersonal skills

Interpersonal skills are crucial to the development of a therapeutic relationship to provide effective nursing care. For qualified nurses this section may help to act as an 'aide-memoire', whilst for those new to nursing it may help to explicate how these skills could be developed. The development of self-awareness is important in terms of learning new interpersonal skills. There is a sense in that having greater self-awareness enables the nurse to use their knowledge and skills to help others (Sully, 2005). Reflection is a fundamental tool in the development of self-awareness; it enables the nurse to make sense of their role in a situation, including the importance of the communication that took place, and to plan how they will provide care and communicate effectively in future (Jasper, 2003).

> **Reflection**
>
> Is there anything you find particularly easy or difficult in communicating with patients and the health and social care team? Why might this be?

Listening

In any exchange between two people it is necessary for one person to listen to another. Listening is essential if communication is to be effective (Burnard, 1998). Active listening is important if practitioners are to demonstrate that they have heard correctly and that they have some insight into what the patient may be feeling. This would seem to be a very elementary statement, but as demonstrated in the earlier research findings, some patients do not feel that they have been listened to adequately (Costa, 2001; Otte, 1996) (Box 2.1).

Box 2.1 The elements of active listening

- Allow the person to speak at their own pace and in their own time
- Thank the person for telling you what they have
- Check you have understood what they are saying:
  - Restate key points in your own words
  - Summarise where the conversation has got to and what you have agreed
  - Ask non-threatening questions
- Reflect on your experience and what you have learnt, and use the new ideas and skills in future dialogues

In any two-way exchange it is better if the individuals involved can relate to each other at the same level, although this may prove difficult in a busy short-stay area. Engaging with another person whilst towering above them does little to foster trust and tends to reinforce the notion of the empowered (health care professional) and the disempowered (patient(s)). Equalising with the level of the patient helps practitioners to engage on a similar level. Simple strategies such as this not only serve to engage the patient in conversation, but may also help prevent or diffuse, aggressive and potentially violent situations. The importance of non-verbal communication (body language) should never be underestimated, as in day-to-day interactions we transmit messages about ourselves not only by the way we walk and the postures we use, but also by the clothes we wear and even the way we wear our hair (Ottenheimer, 2007).

Egan (2002) suggests adopting the following non-verbal body language to help the practitioner demonstrate genuineness and respect towards a patient. This approach is often referred to as using the SOLER position, an acronym developed by Egan to help practitioners to remember the approach (Egan, 2002, pp. 69–70):

S – face the patient Squarely
O – adopt an Open position
L – Lean slightly towards the patient
E – Eye contact
R – Relax

Whilst these may appear to be unrealistic expectations of practitioners working in a busy health care setting, an understanding of how to adopt some of these skills may, nevertheless, help to establish trust in the relationship. Facing the patient squarely sends a powerful message that the practitioner is focused on them. Crossed arms and legs act as barriers and could be avoided. Leaning slightly towards the patient helps to demonstrate a degree of willingness on the part of the practitioner to become involved with the patient. Establishing and maintaining eye contact is important, as this lets the patient know that the practitioner is interested in what is being said to them. Adopting a relaxed posture is more likely to help the patient relax by confirming the practitioner's undivided attention and that they are not likely to suddenly leave for another task or patient.

Central to the notion of listening must be the ability to reflect back to the person talking a sense that they have been actively listened to. There is nothing more frustrating than being asked a question by the person being spoken to about an aspect of the conversation that has already been imparted. There are a number of ways of demonstrating listening to another person's conversation, and some are outlined below in no particular order. These skills, which may at first sight seem to come effortlessly to some practitioners more than others, can easily be learnt. Rehearsing the following methods in a safe environment beforehand, for example whilst socialising with friends, will help the practitioner to learn and become more familiar with these techniques.

Summarising

The technique of summarising helps both the person who is conveying information as well as the listener. Summarising comprises the skill of summing up what has already been discussed and, at intervals during a conversation, reflecting this back to the listener in a few sentences. This is particularly useful, as it not only conveys a sense that the patient has been heard, but also provides an opportunity for a rest during conversation.

This technique also helps those involved in the two-way exchange to gather their thoughts and for the practitioner to check that the patient understands what has been said. It enables the conversation to move on, thereby reducing the likelihood of 'going over old ground'. New topics can be introduced or addressed, if and when the conversation resumes.

Patients are more likely to disclose key pieces of information which may be of concern to them during the use of this technique. However, it is very difficult to know what another person is feeling and the practitioner needs to guard against saying that they know what their patient is going through. It is important that the practitioner does not make assumptions about what the patient is trying to impart on either an informational or a feelings level, but rather that they listen to what the patient is actually saying.

Reflecting back

Reflecting back what the patient has said enables the practitioner to explore feelings that the patient may be experiencing and also to check for accuracy (Beckman Murray and Proctor Zentner, 1989). Demonstrating an ability to do this may help the person who is being listened to feel that the listener has 'captured the moment' and as a result demonstrates a degree of empathy. In other words, the patient has a sense that the practitioner knows 'where they are coming from'. What may be helpful when feelings are being talked about might be the practitioner's ability to capture in a word or two a sense of the feeling behind the words conveyed.

For example an elderly woman in conversation may state that she has felt very alone since her husband died.

Patient: I feel so on my own since Fred died.
Practitioner: . . . you feel lonely?
Patient: Lonely, yes, a lot of the time – but my daughter does pop in twice a week to see that I am OK.

This approach helps to convey a sense of empathy rather than one of sympathy, but also enables the patient to expand on things (Stanton, 2004).

Questioning techniques

There are a number of instances in the therapeutic relationship when the nurse has to ask questions of the patient. Questioning may be mundane, such as questions about the patient's name, marital status, etc., or may be more challenging, such as questions about distressing symptoms or about highly personal or emotive issues. The ability to question thoroughly and sympathetically will enable the nurse to gain a lot of information from the patient, which may help inform the diagnostic and/or therapeutic process.

The following sections explore some of the questioning methods used in the clinical setting and their usefulness.

Open questions

Open questions are particularly useful when helping patients to expand aspects of their conversation. They allow patients to increase topics and demonstrate that the practitioner has time to listen to the responses that the patient may give. For example:

Practitioner: Tell me about the type of pain that you are experiencing.
Practitioner: What worries you about the investigation that you are going to have today?

Open questions are not value-laden; they do not send a message to the recipient that a certain answer is expected or that what they might say is wrong. The description of the symptoms of an illness is best ascertained using open questions, as open questions do not lead the respondent (Kvale, 1996).

Closed questions

Closed questions are useful when practitioners seek to obtain one-word answers, for example when conducting an initial patient assessment.

Practitioner: How old are you? Where do you experience the pain? Who is coming in later to take you home?

Closed questions need to be used carefully, or the patient may feel that the practitioner is rushing and not really willing to hear what they may have to say further on a subject. This is likely if they are concerned about how the practitioner may respond to them when asked a question that the patient feels is difficult to ask.

Using closed questions is also important when engaging with breathless patients for whom a one- or two-word answer may be all they can manage, or respond to, without tiring too much.

Probing questions

The use of probing questions allows the practitioner to further explore responses given by a patient and the patient to expand on what they are saying. For example:

Practitioner: Tell me about the discharge that you get from the wound.
Patient: It soaks through the plaster and wets my clothes.
Practitioner: What do you notice about the colour and smell of the discharge?

Such probing may be useful in the clinical setting when more detail is needed to gain an insight into a patient's condition or when dates are needed in order to establish a diagnosis. Probing also sends the message to the patient that the nurse is interested and wants to know more about them or their condition.

Multiple questions

Multiple questions need to be avoided, if possible, as they tend to confuse patients, and patients usually respond only to the last question of the sentence. For example:

Practitioner: Can you describe your pain, and how long have you had it? Does it come and go or do you have it all the time?
Patient: No, I only get the pain about an hour after eating.

Leading questions

On the whole, leading questions should be avoided as they contain the desired response in the question, even if unwittingly. For example:

Practitioner: Mr Smith's operation is scheduled for at 2 p.m., isn't it?
Colleague: Yes, that's right.

Practitioner: You are in pain at the moment, aren't you Mr Smith?
Mr Smith: 'Yes, I am.

Leading questions can also be patronising or intimidating for those who are receiving them. Because the desired response (either consciously or unconsciously) is delivered in the question, it is difficult for the patient to disagree, and such questions can be very disempowering when used to communicate with those who are deemed most vulnerable in society, for example children and the elderly.

Rhetorical questions

Rhetorical questions are essentially those that require no answer. For example:

Practitioner: It certainly is a bright day today, isn't it?

Learning how to utilise these verbal skills is a fundamental aspect of good quality patient care. Not only is it courteous, but it also potentially impacts on the quality of the therapeutic relationship and as such should not be ignored.

Non-verbal aspects

Whilst the practitioner can learn a lot about their patient when engaging verbally with them, important information is also conveyed non-verbally by the patient and these aspects are often referred to as 'non-verbal cues'. Facial expression, gestures and eye contact help to provide other cues to how the patient may be feeling about the information that is being conveyed to them by the practitioner. The following example helps to highlight these aspects:

> Following surgery the patient may be experiencing pain. This may be directly related to the site of the operation, for example a hernia repair and lower abdominal pain. If the patient conveys this verbally to the practitioner who is looking after them while an inpatient, then medication can be administered to alleviate the pain. The patient may be reluctant to bother the practitioner if they perceive that he/she is busy, and so the pain that the patient is experiencing may go unnoticed.

However, although not conscious of the patient's unreported pain, the skilled practitioner may notice other telltale clues (non-verbal) that lead to suspecting that the patient is in pain. The skilled practitioner may notice that the patient is grimacing or that the patient is holding the part of the body that is hurting.

Further verbal exploration by the practitioner, once this non-verbal cue is noticed, may help them to then respond to the patient and ascertain the problem that the patient is experiencing. This is especially important in vulnerable individuals, for example small children and the elderly, where giving verbal assent to a problem may be more difficult for them and also the practitioner in terms of recognising the message that they are trying to convey.

Patients who, for one reason or another, find it difficult to respond to health care professionals when asked to make decisions about their health care needs rely on the practitioner to support and help them to come to decisions and convey those decisions to other health care professionals. Although this sounds relatively easy, in practice there are times when the decisions made by patients may not sit comfortably with the health care professionals who are looking after them, for example those with learning difficulties or those who by virtue of their reduced capacity to make decisions about their ongoing health care needs. It is at times like these that the patient needs to have someone who will support them in their decision and stand at the interface between them and health care professionals who may be advocating a course of action or intervention that they do not want to follow.

Following an investigation, a patient who has been told that a bowel resection for cancer may add another 5 years to their lifespan may choose to allow nature to take its course and therefore decline further surgical intervention. Although on the surface this may seem a strange decision for a patient to make, in reality this decision may be one of many that the patient has had to make over the past few years and the patient may be tired of fighting their disease and opt to settle for some quality of life in the ensuing days and months.

Clearly, there is a need for some patients to have someone who can 'plead their cause' and who is not afraid to convey the patients' wishes to other health care professionals who are there to look after them. The role of an advocate is an important role for the practitioner and the patient alike although not without its problems, as the practitioner seeks to stand up and speak for the patient in terms of the choices that the patient has come to make and own.

Patient advocacy

Advocacy for, and empowerment of, patients is regarded by many health care professionals as a central tenet of modern health care provision. Much has been written about the nature and purpose of advocacy and empowerment in health care settings (Vaartio et al., 2006; Wheeler, 2000).

This section of the chapter seeks to define what might be meant by empowerment and advocacy in outpatient and day care settings, and how this might be achieved. It further seeks to explore how considerations of advocacy and empowerment might inform health care professionals in their communications with patients.

First it is important to recognise what some commentators mean when they use the terms empowerment and advocacy. It is then necessary to define what is meant by advocacy and empowerment when they are referred to in this book. The nature and ethical justification for advocacy and empowerment may then be considered in order to illuminate why and how these two seemingly different ideas are in fact related, and why they are fundamentally allied to the discussion about the nature of and methods for communicating in the outpatient and day care settings. The discussion therefore links to the role of the health care professionals working in such settings.

The *Oxford English Dictionary* (1989) defines an *advocate* as 'one who pleads the cause of another'. Indeed, most definitions of what it means to act as a patient advocate seem to engender some sort of interpretation of this notion of 'pleading the cause of another'. Advocacy is often assumed by caring professionals to be the act of representing the best interests of the patient; such an interpretation is, however, open to question.

It may be the case that the professional, acting as advocate, is representing the best interests of the patient as explained by the patient to the professional. All too often, however, the term 'acting in the patient's best interest' is heard when professionals have made judgements about patients' care which have not been discussed with them.

Representing the assumed best interests of another supposes that the professional somehow knows what is best for the patient or that the patient is in some way incapable of making decisions for themselves. Such a position is widely reflected in the literature, with commentators observing that patients are vulnerable when caught up in the powerful machinery of the health care system (Copp, 1986); subjected to well-meaning benevolent paternalism (Tuxill, 1994); overawed by bureaucracy, science and technology (Illich, 1977; Weber, 1978). Indeed, Parsons (1951) termed the phrase 'learned helplessness' for this very state.

Representing these assumed best interests further presupposes that the patient is orientated towards what might be called 'medical decisions in the technical sense' (Benjamin and Curtis, 1992, p. 105) when in fact they may be more concerned with what Dworkin (1993, p. 204) calls 'critical interests'. A tangible example of this is when an individual chooses not to have treatment for religious (critical) reasons.

Advocacy is regarded by some as simply representing the views of another to a third party. Dubler (1992, p. 85) defines advocacy within the caring professions as 'acting to the limit of professional ability to provide for the patient's interests and needs as the patient defines them'.

From this standpoint then, a true advocate will put aside their own views and will seek only to represent the point of view of the person they are advocating for. Indeed, this stance is quite close to the true meaning of the word. Such a view may, however, be naïve in that it assumes that the patient is in a position where they can weigh up the facts for themselves and make an informed decision about what to do. It further assumes that the individual is not influenced by some extraneous factors, folklore or misapprehension.

In this book the term *advocacy* is used to mean the state of affairs that arises when a health care professional has discussed the nature, purpose and likely outcomes of a test, procedure or intervention with an individual, that they have ensured that the individual understands the facts and that they are free and able to make a choice about care for themselves.

This definition reflects the humanistic model proposed by Gadow (1980), which counsels that the patient must define what are their best interests and that the role of the advocate is to help the patient to interpret their situation and allow them to decide on the ensuing course of action. The role of the advocate therefore becomes that of representing the outcome of the discussion to other professionals involved in the patient's care. The advocate will act only when the individual patient feels unable or unwilling to represent their view or when the patient is not present when discussion of their care is taking place.

Patient empowerment

This view of advocacy is closely allied to the view of empowerment this book seeks to represent. *Empowerment* is being defined as enabling individuals to speak for themselves when they have been given, and have understood, information regarding their care. It recognises, like advocacy, that most people are both willing and able to make choices about their own lives and health care. It also recognises that some people choose not to exercise this right and that others cannot.

The view of advocacy and empowerment employed in this book also recognises that some people choose to take the advice of the professionals and does not regard this as disempowering. The patient who asks 'what would you do' may be regarded as exercising choice in the same way that many of us do when we take our car for repair or servicing and we ask the mechanic 'what is the best thing to do?'

Empowerment and advocacy might usefully be considered as being part of the same continuum. This continuum recognises the patient as the central point of force of decision making with regard to health care choices. Such a view recognises the individual as both autonomous and capable of understanding, reason and exercising choice.

As such, this view of advocacy and empowerment is a pragmatic one. It recognises that people need information to make choices; they need to understand the information and they need the autonomy to exercise choice. In most cases the exercise of choice will be to follow a route suggested by the professionals because people have made the judgement that this is in their best interests as they see them.

Informed consent

Informed consent is one area where patients are encouraged and supported in making explicit decisions about their health care. Beauchamp and Childress (2001, p. 80) highlight seven elements of informed consent:
Threshold elements (preconditions)

(1) Competence
(2) Voluntariness

Information elements

(3) Disclosure of information
(4) Recommendation
(5) Understanding of information

Consent elements

(6) Decision
(7) Authorisation

Reflecting on these elements, it is plain to see that communication – that is, listening to a patient, information giving and checking that the information has been understood – is fundamental to gaining consent. As with empowerment and advocacy, there is an onus on the professional to ensure that the decisions that the patient takes are voluntary and based on understanding of the information given. Under English law, all adults are deemed competent unless demonstrated otherwise and consent is required for all health care interventions (Mason et al., 2002). In general, verbal consent is sufficient for most procedures, although, plainly, written consent is required for more invasive procedures. The British Department of Health guidance is that:

> it is always best for the person actually treating the patient to seek the patient's consent. However, you may seek consent on behalf of colleagues if you are capable of performing the procedure in question, or if you have been specially trained to seek consent for that procedure(http://www.dh.gov.uk/en/Publicationsandstatistics/Publications/PublicationsPolicyAndGuidance/DH_4006131, no date).

> **Reflection**
>
> Reflect on which of the communication skills discussed in this chapter are important in gaining informed consent from clients.

It is unfortunate that discussions around empowerment and advocacy are still necessary within twenty-first century health care. It may be argued that the need for such discussion may be seen as arising out of an imbalance of power within the health care setting where professionals are seen as all-knowing providers of care and patients are regarded as passive recipients. In some instances, this may be the case; however, even within a more democratic, patient-focused, health care setting the role for advocacy and empowerment may be seen as arising not from misuse of professional power, but as a direct result of the complex nature of health care provision and the fact that professionals are exposed to the language and realities of care on a day-to-day basis, whereas many patients are not.

The role of the outpatient practitioner/student is therefore one that involves communication. As has been seen in this chapter, communication is about a two-way flow of knowledge, ideas, feelings and fears. Communication and the skills it encompasses is the key to providing ethical health care provision. The morally active practitioner will not only understand the different definitions of best interests, but also understand how these might be exercised and protected.

> **Scenario**
> Ms Sophia Jackson, a 28-year-old woman, has come into the unit for a termination of pregnancy. Following a routine admission she is transported to the operating theatre for surgery. Whilst in the anaesthetic room, the nurse looking after her notices that she is beginning to get upset. During questioning it becomes clear that she does not really want to have this termination and says that she is only going through with it as she is afraid of losing her boyfriend.
>
> (1) How may knowledge of interpersonal skills help the nurse to support Sophia at this time?
> (2) What are the wider implications of this scenario in terms of consent?
> (3) What actions may the practitioner take?
>
> Further questioning reveals that her boyfriend has put her under considerable pressure to have the termination and she is not really sure what to do. She thought that she had sorted all this out in her own mind, but is now beginning to have second thoughts.

Summary

The development of day services places considerable demands on health care professionals as they seek to establish a therapeutic relationship with their patients during a shorter period of interaction together. Understanding the difficulties that patients have experienced whilst attending day care settings helps to inform of practice that needs to be adopted to facilitate a better standard of care for both patients and their families and carers. Acquiring and using appropriate interpersonal skills helps practitioners to understand and respond more adequately to their patients' needs and concerns, and plan individualised care. By helping patients to make decisions for themselves, a sense of ownership is obtained for their own health care needs and they are more likely to participate in health-promoting activities. Being able to talk in a meaningful way to patients about their best interests is a cornerstone of high-quality ethical healthcare provision.

Glossary of terms

Advocacy
Pleading the cause of another and/or representing the best interests of the patient(s) in spite of potential opposition

Empowerment
Helping another person to make decisions and choices about their health care

Interpersonal skills
A broad term which encompasses the use of verbal and non-verbal skills to enhance more effective communication

Therapeutic relationship
A helping relationship between a patient and a health care practitioner which is enhanced by the use of interpersonal skills

Websites

Best practice in supported decision making
http://www.dh.gov.uk/en/Publicationsandstatistics/Publications/PublicationsPolicy
AndGuidance/DH_074773

Informed consent
http://www.bma.org.uk/ap.nsf/Content/consenttk2
www.man.ac.uk/rcn/informed consent
www.nhs.uk/nationalplan
www.nmc-uk.org
www.rcn.org.uk

References

Arnold, E. and Undermann Boggs, K. (eds) (2003) *Interpersonal Relationships: Professional Communication Skills for Nurses.* St. Louis, MO: Saunders.

Beauchamp, T. and Childress, J. (2001) *Principles of Biomedical Ethics*, 5th ed. Oxford: Oxford University Press.

Beckman Murray, R. and Proctor Zentner, J. (1989) *Nursing Concepts for Health Promotion.* Hemel Hempstead, Hertfordshire, UK: Prentice Hall.

Benjamin, M. and Curtis, J. (1992) *Ethics in Nursing*, 3rd ed. New York: Oxford University Press.

Burnard, P. (1998) Listening as a personal quality. *Journal of Community Nursing 12*(2), pp. 32–34.

Copp, L.A. (1986) The nurse as advocate for vulnerable persons. *Journal of Advanced Nursing 11*, pp. 255–263.

Costa, M. (2001) The lived preoperative experience of ambulatory surgery patients. *AORN Journal 74*(6), pp. 874–881.

Department of Health (2000) *The NHS Plan*. London: HMSO.

Department of Health (2001) *12 Key Points on Consent: The Law in England* [online]. London: HMSO. Available from: http://www.dh.gov.uk/en/Publichealth/Scientificdevelopmentgeneticsandbioethics/Consent/Consentgeneralinformation/index.htm (accessed 13 September 2007).

Dubler, N.N. (1992) Individual advocacy as a governing principle. *Journal of Case Management 13*, pp. 82–86.

Dworkin, R. (1993) *Life's Dominion: An Argument about Abortion and Euthanasia*. London: HarperCollins.

Egan, G. (2002). *The Skilled Helper: A Problem-Management and Opportunity-Development Approach to Helping*, 7th ed. Pacific Grove, CA: Brooks/Cole.

Gadow, S. (1980) Existential advocacy: philosophical foundation of nursing, in Spicker, S.F. and Gadow, S. (eds) *Nursing, Images and Ideals: Opening Dialogue with the Humanities*. New York: Springer, pp. 79–101.

Illich, I. (1977) *Limits to Medicine. Medical Nemesis: The Exploration of Health*. Marion Boyars, London.

Jasper, M. (2003) *Foundations in Nursing and Health Care: Beginning Reflective Practice (Foundations in Nursing and Health Care)*. Cheltenham, Gloucestershire, UK: Nelson Thornes.

Kvale, S. (1996) *Interviews: An Introduction to Qualitative Research Interviewing*. London: Sage.

Mason, J.K., McCall Smith, R.A. and Laurie, G.T. (2002) *Law and Medical Ethics*, 6th ed. London: Butterworth.

National Health Service Modernisation Agency (2003) *Essence of Care: Patient Focussed Benchmarks for Clinical Governance*. London: Department of Health.

Otte, D. (1996) Patients perspectives and experiences of day case surgery. *Journal of Advanced Nursing 23*(6), pp. 1228–1237.

Ottenheimer, H.J. (2007) *The Anthropology of Language: An Introduction to Linguistic Anthropology*. Kansas: Thomson Wadsworth.

Oxford English Dictionary (1989) Oxford: Oxford University Press.

Parsons, T. (1951) *The Social System*. London: Routledge and Kegan Paul Ltd.

Rogan, F.C. and Timmins, F. (2004) Improving communication in day settings. *Nursing Standard 19*(7), pp. 37–42.

Smeltzer, S. and Bare, B. (2004) *Medical-Surgical Nursing*, 10th ed. Philadelphia: Lippincott.

Stanton, N. (2004) *Mastering Communication*, 4th ed. Basingstoke, Hampshire, England: Palgrave MacMillan.

Stein-Parbury, J. (2000) *Patient and person: Developing Interpersonal Skills in Nursing*, 2nd ed. Sydney,: Harcourt.

Sully, P. (2005) Communication in adult nursing, in Brooker, C. and Nicol, M. (eds) *Nursing Adults: The Practice of Caring*. Edinburgh, Midlothian, UK: Mosby, pp. 39–56.

Sully, P. and Dallas, J. (2005) *Essential Communication Skills for Nursing*. Edinburgh, Midlothian, UK: Elsevier/Mosby.

Tuxill, C. (1994) Ethical aspects of critical care, in Millar, B. and Burnard, P. (eds) *Critical Care Nursing: Caring for Critically Ill Adults*. London: Balliere Tindall, pp. 250–272.

Vaartio, H., Leino-Kilpi, H., Salantera, S. and Suominen, T. (2006) Nursing advocacy: how is it defined by patients and nurses, what does it involve and how is it experienced? *Scandinavian Journal of Caring Sciences* 20(3), pp. 282–292.

Weber, M. (1978) *Economy and Society: An Outline of Interpretative Sociology*. California: University of California Press.

Wheeler, P. (2000) Is advocacy at the heart of professional practice? *Nursing Standard* 14(36), pp. 39–41.

Chapter 3

The development of outpatient and day services in primary care

Sarah Pye and Judith Parsons

Learning objectives

(1) Understand recent policy initiatives that have an impact on day services and outpatient clinics
(2) Identify the importance of collaborative working to support the integration of services and continuity of patient care
(3) Explore current provision and future developments in primary care that affect day services and outpatients
(4) Consider the range of treatments available in primary care

Introduction

Definition

Primary care describes the health services that are provided in the local community such as family doctors/general practitioners (GPs), nurses, pharmacists, dentists and midwives. Services include a range of rehabilitation, out-of-hour care, district nursing, occupational health nursing, health visiting and school nursing,

Of all patients receiving health care in the United Kingdom, only 20% are looked after by hospital consultants; the remaining 80% are treated in primary care by GPs and their teams. Doctors and nurses in general practice undertake over 300 million consultations per year (Department of Health (DH), 2007a). With approximately 90% of all patient journeys beginning and ending in primary care, it is perhaps not surprising that recent health care policy is concentrated on improving and increasing activity in this setting. With the first White Paper of the current United Kingdom (UK) Labour government *The New NHS, Modern, Dependable* (DH, 1997) setting the direction, policy has continued to follow this path and the government set out its plans to shift the focus from acute to primary care in 2001 (DH, 2001a). Nurses in primary care have been viewed as central in the achievement of delivering this huge agenda with publications such as 'Liberating the Talents' (DH, 2002a) outlining key roles for nurses. *Modernising Nursing Careers* (DH, 2006a) identifies nurses working in a range of settings, across primary and secondary care. This signifies a move away from traditional career pathways. Nursing careers will no longer be constrained by setting or discipline, but tailored to patient need and follow patient pathways.

Much of the government's reform has been focused on acute hospitals (King Fund, 2006); however, in 2006 the government turned its attention to the community and primary care (DH, 2006b). The shift of the modernisation agenda to primary care has increased the need for collaboration between hospitals and primary care. The current strategy for health care policy is to deliver as much care as possible close to the patient's home, offering easier access, choice and development of a truly patient-led National Health Service (NHS) (DH, 2005a). Services available in primary care began to expand in 2000. The NHS plan (DH, 2000) outlined new roles for GPs. With additional training, GPs would develop expertise in specialist areas of clinical practice such as dermatology and endoscopy. This would enable referrals to be made by other practitioners for patients who would traditionally be referred to a secondary care consultant. These initiatives aim to bring care closer to patients and reduce the demand for hospital services, providing choice and improving access for patients. This may mean fewer beds are needed in acute hospitals.

To demonstrate its commitment to expanding services available in primary care, the government announced major investment to extend the range of services available outside hospital settings (DH, 2006b). Further to this, in the summer of 2007, the Health Minister Professor Ara Darzi began a review of NHS services. The interim report (DH 2007e) proposes further developments for primary care in England, the final report detailing the way forward is expected in the summer of 2008. The shift of services from acute to primary care is a challenge and requires changes in the management of patient care in order to succeed. Communication and collaboration between health professionals across acute and primary care are vital in order to support continuity of patient care. Indeed, in a report commissioned by the government to advise on hospital outpatient services, patient's views were sought; the report commented that patients considered liaison with primary care important (Clinical Standards Advisory Group, 2000).

Checkpoint

What are the principle reasons for the transfer of care from acute hospitals to primary care?

This chapter considers developments in health care and how they have increased the range of services available to patients in their own homes or in alternative settings. It considers the importance of interagency and inter-professional collaboration in the maintenance of an efficient patient journey through the health care system. The role of nurses in the development of primary care services is discussed in relation to day and outpatient services. The potential risks associated with the transfer of care from acute to primary care are also considered.

Reducing the demand for hospital-based services

Developments in primary care mean many patients no longer have to travel to the acute hospital for operations that can be performed as a day case. Outpatient services are increasingly available in the community setting. Patients requiring rehabilitation and management of exacerbations of long-term conditions can receive hospital-type care in their own homes. Intermediate care initiatives include the expansion of bed-based and non-bed-based rehabilitation (see Chapter 12 for examples of these). More patients are now receiving rehabilitation in day hospitals and in their own homes as a result of initial guidance on the development of intermediate care services in 2001 (DH, 2001b). Cancer patients in some areas do not have to go to hospital to receive chemotherapy. All these services are reducing the demand for beds and services in acute hospital settings.

Reflection

Reflect on the likely consequences for care of transferring services into primary care?

General practitioners with a special interest (GPwSI), *pharmacists with a special interest* (PhwSI) and *practitioners with a special interest* (PwSI) (including nurses and allied health professionals) have become specialists in certain clinical areas such as dermatology, orthopaedics and vascular care. Patients can be referred to a GPwSI or PwSI as an alternative to a consultant in a particular specialist field. For nurses the term PwSI does not feature in the publication *Modernising Nursing Careers* (DH, 2006a). However, the publication speaks of nurse specialists, nurse consultants and modern and community matrons. GPwSI deliver services that extend their role of generalists; however, they will not replace hospital consultants (Royal College of General Practitioners, 2002). Guidance to support the implementation of services and accreditation of GPwSI and PhwSI (DH, 2007b) provides practical support to those organisations involved in commissioning to provide care closer to home. The publication also provides some useful case studies. An evaluation of dermatology services undertaken by GPwSI reveals similar clinical outcomes as hospital-based outpatients but was preferred by patients and found to be more accessible (Salisbury et al., 2005). The Australian experience of GPs developing specialist interests provides a note of caution (Wilkinson et al., 2005). There is a concern from Australia that services could become fragmented, and fewer GPs could be working in generalist roles. The disadvantages to patients have been identified as fewer GPs, a lack of communication between practitioners and a lower standard of care.

Opportunity for the student

Are there any GPwSI or PwSI in your locality? What specialities are being developed?

Outcomes from the UK experience are mixed. Evidence suggests that GPwSI provide high-quality care with good clinical outcomes, care is more accessible than hospital outpatient care and waiting times are shorter. There does, however, appear to be some inconsistency in relation to monitoring GPwSI services and models differ (National Co-Ordinating Centre for NHS Service Delivery and Organisation Research and Development (NCCSDO), 2007). The NCCSDO suggests that further research is required.

Minor surgery can also be undertaken in a GP practice, initially enabled by the GP contract in 1990. Since then the number of patients receiving minor surgery in primary care has continued to increase. Although there are potential benefits, there has been little impact on hospital waiting times (NCCSDO, 2007). This could suggest that minor surgery in primary care is not reducing the demand on hospital-based services. Details of the commissioning process and accreditation of GPwSI and PhwSI have been outlined in parts 2 and 3 of *New Guidance – Implementing Care Closer To Home: Convenient Quality Care For Patients* (DH, 2007b).

The expansion of community hospitals could also help realise the aim of care closer to home. It is envisaged that community hospitals could develop a wide range of services traditionally provided in acute hospitals. *Our Health, Our Care, Our Community – Investing in the Future of Community Hospitals and Services* (DH, 2006c) outlines the type of services that could be available for local communities in smaller community hospitals. The type of services that may be provided in this type of setting range from minor injury units to end-of-life care, caring for children and older people. The extent to which services such as these will develop remains to be seen.

Certain assumptions in relation to the transfer of services from acute hospitals to the community have been outlined by the NCCSDO (2007) and are summarised below.

Assumption	Comment
Care can safely be transferred from specialists to primary care practitioners	Not true of minor surgery and not necessarily true of GPSI services
Care in the community is cheaper than care in hospitals	Often not the case. Cost evaluation should not focus purely on NHS costs but also on prices charged by providers
Transferring care into the community will not increase overall demand	There is a serious risk that increasing provision may increase demand either because of increased demand from patients or because of increased referral from GPs
Care in the community is popular with patients and should therefore be encouraged	The general popularity of this policy would not necessarily survive loss of quality and efficiency

Professor Martin Roland, National Primary Care Research and Development Centre, University of Manchester. Reproduced with kind permission of the SDO Programme.

Treatment centres (TC) are an alternative to acute hospital care for patients requiring diagnostic tests and surgery that can be performed as a day case. The aims of the TC are to increase capacity for non-urgent surgery and diagnostic tests and provide an alternative choice for patients. Indeed, the first TCs were set up to help increase capacity and reduce waiting times for specialities such as ophthalmology and orthopaedics. The TC can be described as a unit that provides scheduled (planned) care for NHS patients; they may be run by the NHS or commissioned by primary care trusts from independent companies. The development of the independent sector (IS) TC has increased capacity for day surgery and the performance of diagnostic tests. Further information about TC can be found on the DH website listed at the end of this chapter (DH, 2007c).

Current government policy is committed to develop a patient-led NHS with more and more opportunities available to non-NHS providers. There have been concerns raised in relation to the ISTC. These relate to the possible negative impact on NHS hospitals and on community services (Parish and Learner, 2006; Wallace, 2006). They claim that in some cases the NHS is 'left to pick up the pieces when things go wrong'. There is also a concern that the independent sector providers will choose to undertake simple procedures, leaving the NHS to deal with the more complex cases, which increase the time of patient's stay in acute hospitals. Generally, there is a concern that the ISTC might have a negative effect on the wider health economy. The House of Commons Health Committee (HCHC, 2006) in its report on the ISTC in part has echoed this view. The report concludes that the ISTC does not necessarily offer better care than the NHS. Increasing capacity and the fall in waiting times, the committee considers, could be the result of increased spending generally and again not exclusively due to the ISTC.

Opportunity for the student

Is there a treatment centre in your locality? If so, which organisation is it run by?

Although *practice-based commissioning* (PBC) and *payment by results* (PbR) support the agenda, on choice they have the potential to fragment care by affording the opportunity to many organisations to provide care in the community. Safeguarding the quality of patient care must be the principal aim. The shift from acute hospital-based services to primary care, it would appear, is not without risk (Snow, 2007). Expansion of service providers requires caution. In a speech, Patricia Hewitt (2007) recognises the opportunities, uncertainties and challenges of commissioning new providers. Alternative providers, however, either NHS or non-NHS, will all play a part in the development of primary care services in striving to reduce the demand for hospital-based services. Colin-Thomé (DH, 2007a) envisages 'services for patients outside hospital will be unrecognisable in 10 years'. With services potentially being provided by a number of organisations the need for collaboration is ever more present.

Reflection

What are the strengths and weaknesses of health care being provided by non-NHS providers?

Collaboration

Much has been written about the importance of effective collaboration and communication in health and social care (Barr 2002; Freeth et al., 2002; Meads and Ashcroft, 2005). In developing a new approach to service provision, it is vital to ensure that the patient experiences a seamless journey rather than a series of fragmented episodes of care (DH, 2005a). Health and social care practitioners will need to become effective partners in order to deliver care in new and innovative ways; this will mean a change in practice for many.

The idea of working collaboratively is not new; the language used may be different with the earlier literature often referring to teamworking. In 1988 the World Health Organization (WHO) identified that collaborative working could have a positive effect on health outcomes; since then there has been an increasing body of literature identifying the need for collaboration and inter-professional working (Freeth et al., 2002).

The type of knowledge and skills that are required to work collaboratively, and with more joined up thinking, centres around understanding one's own role and that of others as well as engaging in effective communication. Parsons (in

Colyer and Parsons, 2005) found in a study that all these attributes were evident in inter-professional teams that described themselves as functioning in a collaborative manner. These attributes were expanded to include respect for individuals and their roles and trust amongst team members. Those teams that did not collaborate effectively tended to cite professional rivalry and overwork as reasons for their lack of collaboration.

There is no place for professional rivalries in the provision of health care in the UK today. As has been seen the provision of health care is changing, and roles and responsibilities have altered. For example, once the domain of doctors, prescribing can now be undertaken by nurses, pharmacists and some allied health professionals (DH, 2002b, 2005b, c, 2006e). Effective collaboration can be seen to improve patient outcomes (Meads and Ashcroft, 2005). This would seem to be particularly important when many organisations may be involved in providing care for one patient.

It would appear that as well as skills in collaboration, there needs to be a robust system for sharing information. The single assessment process (SAP) is an example of how information can be shared. It was first highlighted in the *National Service Framework for Older People* (DH, 2001c). It provides an opportunity to access up-to-date information from a range of health and social care professionals, thereby reducing the need for all professionals involved to ask intrusive, repetitive questions of patients. Information is easily accessible and can be shared across organisations and professional disciplines.

For this process to be successful, it seems there has to be a certain reliance on information technology and the compatibility of systems so that information is shared effectively. The principles of the SAP are sound and support collaborative practice. Another example of a framework for sharing information currently being introduced is the *Common Assessment Framework* for children and families (Department for Education and Skills, 2006). Both these examples could be explored when considering how information is shared across organisations providing outpatient and day care services in primary care. The introduction of the new NHS care record system will make sharing and access to information easier, thus increasing communication and collaboration.

Reflection

In what settings, and what format, have you seen patient records? What seemed to work and why?

Treating patients in their own homes

The range of treatments available for patients in their own homes is increasing. Policy makers are determined to ensure that as many people as possible receive treatment, previously only available in hospitals, in their own homes (DH, 2006b). The majority of that care is being provided by nurses in partnership with other health and social care practitioners (DH, 2002a). The DH has created a toolkit for disease management to inform both service providers in primary and secondary care and the primary care commissioners of these services (DH, 2007d). In England 15 million people report that they have long-term conditions and 5% of patients mainly those with long-term conditions account for 42% of all acute bed occupancy (DH, 2007d). In order to provide a range of new services in primary care new roles have been created to deliver them (DH, 2004a).

The community matron role is discussed in a document called *Supporting People with Long Term Conditions: Liberating the talents of nurses who care for people with long-term conditions* (DH, 2005d). The title is interesting in that it suggests, as did the former document (DH, 2002a), that community nurses have not necessarily been working in the most effective ways to enable them to use their existing skills. By building on their current knowledge and skills nurses are in a prime position to work with people who suffer from long-term conditions and who it is seen put the most pressure on secondary care services (DH, 2005d). In order to deal with this the community matron role has been created to enable experienced nurses to use case management to reduce the number of 'frequent fliers', people with long-term conditions who are frequently readmitted to hospital because of an exacerbation or crisis with their disease management. These community matrons provide intensive help to these patients to enable them to remain at home longer, providing them more choice about their health care. By using case management skills they are able to work collaboratively across primary and secondary care and with other agencies, such as social services, to stabilise patients and maintain them in their own homes.

It has been proposed that as a result of improved management, emergency bed usage will be reduced by 5% by 2008 (DH, 2005d). This model of care is based on two schemes that were used in the USA, 'Evercare' and 'Kaiser Permanente'. Figure 3.1 shows the role of the community matron in case management working with people with highly complex long-term conditions at level 3. The type of skills which community nurses need to be proficient in can be found in the chief nurse's list of ten key roles (DH, 2002a) that are listed later in this chapter.

Opportunity for the student

Which of the ten key roles do you think community matrons will need to carry out their role effectively? (see the section 'Future directions' for the ten key roles.)

It has been suggested that some of the nurses with the best skills to develop as community matrons are district nurses (DH, 2005d). This is because they already hold a post-registration community specialist practice qualification normally at undergraduate level and have the working knowledge of primary and community care. Nurses from secondary care may have some of the clinical skills to work with people with long-term conditions, but will be required to undertake further education to orientate them to working in primary care (DH, 2005a). This reflects the more recent suggestion found in *Modernising Nursing Careers* (DH, 2006a), which proposes that nurses need to be more flexible and follow careers based on patient pathways.

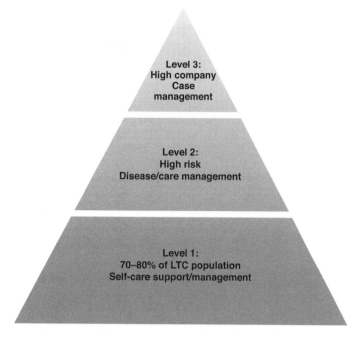

Figure 3.1   The Kaiser Permanente triangle [DH, 2005c, reproduced under the terms of the Click-Use Licence].

Nurses are also working in new ways in general practice where practice nurses work in collaboration with GPs to help to deliver the standards for quality outcomes framework (DH, 2004a). Much of this work consists of working with patients in helping them maintain their long-term conditions, but at levels 1 and 2 of the Kaiser Permanente triangle (see Figure 3.1) with a different level of patient to the community matron. Firstly, these groups are normally sufficiently mobile to attend a GP practice, and secondly, much of the work carried out by the practice nurse is based on the best practice identified in the quality outcomes framework, which is based on the National Service Frameworks. In addition, a public health approach of working with people to prevent disease is used to collaborate with patients to prevent further deterioration in their conditions. This may mean patients taking more control of their condition and move from a level 2 to a level 1, or be better controlled at level 2 (see Figure 3.1).

The type of patient groups commonly managed in this way in general practice include people with diabetes, asthma, chronic obstructive pulmonary disease, renal disease and coronary heart disease. Therefore, many of these patients will never attend outpatient clinics; if they require medical input, they are likely to be managed by a GPwSI. An additional area of support for people with long-term conditions is the expert patient programme (DH, 2001d), which recognises patients as key decision makers in their care and often more expert in their individual situation than the health care professionals who care for them. There is provision available for patients to attend programmes which are expert patient led to facilitate their understanding and management of their condition. All these approaches can be seen to be meeting the requirements of *Our Health, Our Care, Our Say* (DH, 2006b), which showed that people wanted to be treated faster in more familiar surroundings closer to their homes.

Telephone triage is another example of nurses taking on new roles and is used in out-of-hour services, general practice and NHS Direct (Richards et al., 2004). The purpose of triage is to make decisions about what the level of patient need is and which professional is best skilled to intervene to support them. The support may be advice given on issues like basic home first aid, or self-medication, to buying an over-the-counter medicine, or seeking the advice of a pharmacist, to being seen by a practice nurse, nurse practitioner or GP, to being sent to the nearest accident and emergency department, or minor injuries unit. Telephone triage has been in use since the 1990s, but a newer intervention is telemedicine. This allows nurses or doctors to talk directly with their patients, download and monitor observations such as blood pressure levels and change treatment. Again, these new approaches to care delivery provide the patient with care within their own home and prevent long trips to out-patients departments and appear to have successful outcomes (Clark et al., 2007).

District nurses have provided care in peoples' homes since the middle of the nineteenth century. Today they continue in this role, albeit as leaders of a team, and they have taken on many activities that were normally carried out in secondary care. This includes intravenous antibiotic therapy (Corwin et al., 2005), chemotherapy (Nursing Standard News, 2005) and blood transfusions (Audit Commission, 1999). The advantage of developing these services means that patients can remain at home or attend a nurse-led clinic very close to their home.

Reflection

Reflect on the pros and cons of the provision of these services at home.

Alongside these moves towards more primary care, provision of services is the subsequent reduction in secondary care provision. The rate at which this happens has varied nationally and is based on the priorities the former primary care trusts gave to delivering these services. In most instances they will have been based on a health needs assessment (Cavanagh and Chadwick, 2005), which identifies the health needs of the local population and then plans services to meet those needs. With the development of primary-care-led services and practice-based commissioning more services are likely to be commissioned in the private sector (Lewis et al., 2007), but are still likely to be delivered closer to patients' homes and more nurses can expect to be practising in primary care (DH, 2006a).

Future directions

What does the expansion of services in primary care mean for the future of the NHS and the role of nurses? Earlier in the chapter it was noted that the increased demand for day surgery increases the need for health and social care provision in the community. It was identified that the move from acute hospital-based outpatients and day services is not without risk. The challenge is to ensure services are safe and quality of care is maintained. *Standards for Better Health* (DH, 2004b) apply to all services provided within the NHS and the independent sector and should be referred to during the commissioning process of all health care services. The ability to collaborate with a multitude of organisations and health care professionals within these organisations is fundamental to safe, effective patient care. Nurses could play a key role in the delivery of care closer to home. The changing role of the community nurse first outlined by the DH in *Liberating The Talent'* (DH, 2002a) identified ten key roles for community nurses:

- To order diagnostic investigations such as pathology test and X-rays
- To make and receive referrals direct, say, to a therapist or pain consultants
- To admit and discharge patients for specified conditions and within agreed protocols
- To manage patient caseloads, say, for diabetes or rheumatology
- To run clinics, say, for ophthalmology or dermatology
- To prescribe medicines and treatments
- To carry out a wide range of resuscitation procedures including defibrillation
- To perform minor surgery and outpatient procedures
- To triage patients using the latest IT to be seen by the most appropriate health professional
- To take the lead in the way local health services are organised and the way that they are run

The development of these roles is essential to the transfer of outpatient and day services to the community. The direction this publication sets for community nursing has continued. More recently, the DH (2006a) has clearly identified the actions required from nurses, employers and those involved in nurse education to deliver the 'Care Closer to Home' agenda. Nurse education, both pre- and post-registration, needs to reflect the changing environments in which nurses will work.

Community nurses are in a privileged position to hear and respond to the patient voice, making sure services are developed in a truly patient-centred way. Involvement in commissioning is important for nurses. Their clinical knowledge, awareness of health need and health promotion and the ability to negotiate across different professional groups and with the public are all important skills in commissioning (Kaufman, 2002). Nurses will need leadership and entrepreneurial skills in order to ensure that they are involved in the development of services to meet patient need. PBC will provide opportunities for nurses to be involved in the commissioning process, helping to redesign services around the needs of local populations (Dilks, 2006). Nurses of the future will require skills in advanced practice, enabling them to respond to the agenda on choice and the changing roles of other health care practitioners, such as GPs. Although there have been many changes, and indeed many more to come, in the way services are delivered the core functions of community nurses identified remain essential for community nursing in the future (DH, 2002a).

Opportunity for the student

Try and find out what involvement nurses have locally in commissioning services.

Skills in health education and health promotion are fundamental to ensuring that patients remain safe in their own homes (Chilton et al., 2004; Hyde, 2001). The 'Choose and Book' initiative is an example of the need for health information for patients. With a choice of providers, patients need to understand the risks and benefits of differences in waiting times for example and be choosing the best option for them fully informed of potential risks and benefits to their health. Patients with long-term conditions managing acute exacerbations of their condition at home need to have an understanding of their condition, how to access support quickly and be confident in the skills and knowledge of the nurses caring for them during times of acute illness.

Reflection

What skills have you already developed that might translate into working in community-based services?

Despite the shift from acute hospital care to community care there has been a dramatic fall in the number of places on district nursing courses, with some universities cutting the course altogether (Harrison, 2006). The drive to shift care from acute hospitals to primary care means that increasing numbers of newly qualified nurses will start their careers in the community (DH, 2006a). With decreasing numbers of qualified district nurses there could be a danger that experienced nurses will not be available in required numbers to support these newly qualified staff nurses in the community setting. Nurses will need to be equipped to work with diverse groups of people in a variety of settings. For high-quality care closer to home preregistration training should recognise the changing environments nurses will work in and provide a stronger focus on the community. It may be that a more generalist approach is needed and nurses are no longer educated within the current branch system (Snow, 2006). This is currently one of the options being considered by the NMC for pre-registration training.

Scenario

Mr Peter Jones is a 46-year-old gentleman who has a 4-month history of shortness of breath when climbing a flight of stairs. He has recently given up smoking and is suffering with an irritating morning cough. He has been to see his GP who has referred him to the nurse practitioner who has a special interest in respiratory disease.

(1) What developments in primary care have enabled this referral?
(2) Which of the ten key roles identified for community nurses are particularly important for the nurse practitioner in this case?
(3) What other skills and knowledge identified in this chapter will the nurse practitioner use?
(4) Who will the nurse practitioner need to collaborate with to provide efficient, effective, safe care for this patient?

Summary

The drive to focus health services closer to patients is undoubtedly a challenge. Many changes to the health care system have already been implemented to facilitate the move. Patients have a choice in where they access some elements of their health care. The service provision in primary care is increasing and the demand for acute hospital-based services reducing. Benefits for patients should be the basis on which decisions are made and where risks are identified cohesive steps with all organisations involved taken to minimise them to ensure patient safety. There will unquestionably be more challenges along the way but also many opportunities to develop a health service that is safe, effective, responsive, flexible and, importantly, one that patients have been involved in developing and that they have confidence in.

Glossary of terms

General practitioners with a special interest (GPwSI)

A general practitioner who has undergone additional training in a specialist clinical field, e.g. dermatology

Payment by results (PbR)

The tariff-based payment system for providers of care to NHS patients, based on the activity undertaken

Pharmacists with a special interest (PhwSI)

A pharmacist who has undergone additional training in a specialist clinical field, e.g. asthma

Practice-based commissioning (PBC)

Commissioning of local health services by a group of general practitioners

Practitioners with a special interest (PwSI)

A health professional (nurse or physiotherapist) who has undergone additional training in a specialist clinical field

Treatment centres (TC)

Treatment centres are units that offering, pre-booked day and short-stay surgery and diagnostic procedures

Websites

www.dh.gov.uk
www.institute.nhs.uk
www.improvementfoundation.org
www.kingsfund.org.uk
www.primarycarecontracting.nhs.uk
www.nhscarerecords.nhs.uk
www.ournhs.nhs.uk/

References

Audit Commission (1999) *First Assessment: A Review of District Nursing Services in England and Wales.* London: Audit Commission Publications.

Barr, H. (2002) *Interprofessional Education: Today, Yesterday and Tomorrow.* Occasional Paper No 1. Learning and Teaching Support Network for Health Science and Practice. London: Kings College.

Cavanagh, S. and Chadwick, K. (2005) *Health Needs Assessment: A Practical Guide.* London: National Institute for Health and Clinical Excellence.

Chilton, S., Melling, K., Drew, D. and Clarridge, A. (2004) *Nursing in the Community.* London: Arnold.

Clark, R.A., Inglis, S.C., McAlister, F.A., Cleland, J.G.F. and Stewart, S. (2007) Telemonitoring or structured telephone support programmes for patients with chronic heart failure: systematic review and meta-analysis. *BMJ 334,* p. 942.

Clinical Standards Advisory Group (2000) *A Study of Hospital Outpatient Services Report of a CSAG Committee Chaired by Professor Pamela Enderby* [online]. Available from: http://www.dh.gov.uk/assetRoot/04/01/45/52/04014552.pdf (accessed 10 June 2007).

Colyer, H. and Parsons, J. (2005) *Modernising Pre-registration Education for the Allied Health Professions. First Wave Development Funded Project 2002–2005.* Report to the Department of Health. London: Department of Health.

Corwin, P., Toop, L., McGeoch, G., Than, M., Wynn-Thomas, S., Well, E.J., Dawson, R., Abernethy, P., Pithie, A., Chamber, S., Fletcher, L. and Richards, D. (2005) Randomised control trial of IV antibiotics for cellulitis at home compared with hospital. *BMJ 330*(7483): 129.

Dilks, S. (2006) Buying for results. *Nursing Standard 20*(29), pp. 70–71.

Freeth, D., Hammick, M., Barr, H., Koppel, I. and Reeves, S. (2002) *A Critical Review of Evaluations of Interprofessional Education.* Occasional Paper No 2. Learning and Teaching Support Network for Health Science and Practice. London: Kings College London.

Department of Education and Skills (2006) *Common Assessment Framework.* London: Stationery Office.

Department of Health (DH) (1997) *The New NHS: Modern, Dependable.* London: Stationery Office.

Department of Health (DH) (2000) *The NHS Plan.* London: Stationery Office.

Department of Health (DH) (2001a) *Shifting the Balance of Power Within the NHS: Securing Delivery* [online]. Available from: http://www.dh.gov.uk/en/Publicationsandstatistics/Publications/PublicationsPolicyAndGuidance/DN_4009844 (accessed 10 June 2007).

Department of Health (DH) (2001b) *Intermediate Care: Local Authority Circular* (2001)1 [online]. Available from: http://www.dh.gov.uk/en/Publicationsandstatistics/Lettersandcirculars/LocalAuthority
Circulars/AllLocalAuthority/DH_4003698 (accessed 10 June 2007).

Department of Health (DH) (2001c) *National Service Framework for Older People.* London: Stationery Office.

Department of Health (DH) (2001d) *The Expert Patient.* London: Stationery Office.

Department of Health (DH) (2002a) *Liberating the Talents: Helping Primary Care Trusts and Nurses to Deliver the NHS Plan.* London: Stationery Office.

Department of Health (DH) (2002b) Press Release: *Groundbreaking New Consultation Aims to Extend Prescribing Powers for Pharmacists and Nurses* [online]. Available from: http://www.dh.gov.uk/en/Publicationsandstatistics/Pressreleases/DH_4013114 (accessed 10 June 2007).

Department of Health (DH) (2004a) *Updated Version of Original QOF Guidance and Evidence Base* [online]. Available from: http://www.dh.gov.uk/en/Healthcare/ Primarycare/Primarycarecontracting/QOF/DH_4125653 (accessed 10 June 2007).

Department of Health (DH) (2004b) *Standards for Better Health.* London: Stationery Office.

Department of Health (DH) (2005a) *Commissioning a Patient-Led NHS* [online]. Available from: http://www.dh.gov.uk/en/Publicationsandstatistics/Publications/PublicationsPolicy AndGuidance/DH_4116716 (accessed 10 June 2007).

Department of Health (DH) (2005b) *Summary of Changes to Regulations on Supplementary Prescribing – April 2005* [online]. Available from: http://www.dh.gov.uk/ en/Policyandguidance/Medicinespharmacyandindustry/Prescriptions/TheNon-Medical PrescribingProgramme/Supplementaryprescribing/DH_4123024 (accessed 10 June 2007).

Department of Health (DH) (2005c) Press Release: *Nurse and Pharmacist Prescribing Powers Extended* [online]. Available from: http://www.dh.gov.uk/en/Healthcare/ Medicinespharmacyandindustry/Prescriptions/TheNon-MedicalPrescribingProgramme/ Supplementaryprescribing/DH_4123024 (accessed 10 June 2007).

Department of Health (DH) (2005d) *Supporting People with Long Term Conditions: Liberating the Talents of Nurses Who Care for People with Long-Term Conditions.* London: Stationery Office.

Department of Health – CNO's Directorate (2006a) *Modernising Nursing Careers Setting the Direction.* London: Stationery Office.

Department of Health (DH) (2006b) *Our Health, Our Care, Our Say: A New Direction for Community Services.* London: Stationery Office.

Department of Health (DH) (2006c) *Our Health, Our Care, Our Community – Investing in the Future of Community Hospitals and Services.* London: The Stationery Office.

Department of Health (DH) (2006d) *Tackling Hospital Waiting: The 18 Week Patient Pathway: An Implementation Framework.* London: Stationery Office.

Department of Health (DH) (2006e) *Improving Patients' Access to Medicines: A Guide to Implementing Nurse and Pharmacist Independent Prescribing Within the NHS.* London: Stationery Office.

Department of Health (DH) (2007a) *Keeping it Personal Clinical Case for Change: Report by David Colin-Thomé, National Director for Primary Care* [online]. Available from: http://www.dh.gov.uk/en/Publicationsandstatistics/Publications/PublicationsPolicyAnd Guidance/DH_065094 (accessed 10 June 2007).

Department of Health (DH) (2007b) *New Guidance – Implementing Care Closer to Home: Convenient Quality Care for Patients.* London: Department of Health [online]. Available from: http://www.dh.gov.uk/en/Healthcare/Primarycare/Practitionerswithspecialinterests/DH_074419 (accessed 10 June 2007).

Department of Health (DH) (2007c) *Treatment Centres* [online]. Available from: http://www.dh.gov.uk/en/Healthcare/Primarycare/Treatmentcentres/index.htm (accessed 10 June 2007).

Department of Health (DH) (2007d) *Disease Management Information Toolkit (DIMT).* London: Stationery Office.

Department of Health (2007e) Our NHS Our Future. NHS next stage review interim report. London Department of Heath [on-line]. Available from: http://www.oumhs. nhs.uk/fromtypepad/2834n_OurNHS_r3acc.pdf (accessed 1/11/07)

Harrison, S. (2006) Changing role is blamed for cuts to district nurse training courses. *Nursing Standard 20*(38), p. 6.

Hewitt, P. (2007) *Speech by Rt Hon Patricia Hewitt MP, Secretary of State for Health, 20 February 2007 to the King's Fund: Commissioning New Providers* [online]. Available from: http://www.dh.gov.uk/en/News/Speeches/DH_074569 (accessed 10 June 2007).

House of Commons Health Committee (2006) *Independent Sector Treatment Centres Fourth Report of Session 2005–06*, Vol. I. London: House of Commons Health Committee.

Hyde, V. (2001) *Community Nursing and Health Care Insights and Innovations*. London: Arnold.

Kaufman, G. (2002) Investigating the nursing contribution to commissioning in primary health-care. *Journal of Nursing Management 10*(2), pp. 83–94.

King Fund (2006) *Kings Fund Briefing. Our Health, Our Care, Our Say: A New Direction for Community services*. London: Kings Fund.

Lewis, R., Curry, N. and Dixon, M. (2007) *Practice Based Commissioning: From Good Idea to Effective Practice*. London: The Kings Fund.

Meads, G. and Ashcroft, J. (2005) *The Case for Interprofessional Collaboration*. Oxford: Blackwell Publiishing/CAIPE.

National Co-Ordinating Centre for NHS Service Delivery and Organisation Research and Development (2007) *Can Primary Care Reform Reduce Demand on Hospital Outpatient Departments?* [online]. Available from: http://www.sdo.lshtm.ac.uk/files/adhoc/82-research-summary.pdf (accessed 10 June 2007).

Nursing Standard News (2005) Home chemotherapy to be expanded. *Nursing Standard 19*(22), p. 8.

Parish, C. and Learner, S. (2006) A private war in the NHS. *Nursing Standard 20*(32), pp. 14–16.

Richards, D.A., Meakins, J., Tarofik, J., Godfrey, L., Dutton, E. and Heywood, P. (2004) Quality monitoring of nurse telephone triage. *Journal of Advanced Nursing 47*(5), pp. 551–560.

Royal College of General Practitioners (2002) *Implementing a Scheme for General Practitioners*. London: Department of Health and Royal College of General Practitioners.

Salisbury, C., Noble, A., Horrocks, S., Crosby, Z., Harrison, V., Coast, J., Berker, D. and Peters, T. (2005) Evaluation of a general practitioner with special interest service for dermatology: randomised controlled trial. *British Medical Journal 331*(7530), 1441.

Snow, T. (2006) Training faces biggest shake-up since project 2000. *Nursing Standard 21*(1), pp. 12–13.

Snow, T. (2007) In the balance: the shift from hospitals into the community *Nursing Standard 21*(34), pp. 12–13.

Wilkinson, D., Dick, M. and Askew, D. (2005) General practitioners with special interests: risk of a good thing becoming bad? *Medical Journal of Australia 183*(2), pp. 84–86 [online]. Available from: http://mja.com.au/public/issues/183_02_180705/wil10365_fm.html (accessed 10 June 2007).

Wallace, A. (March 2006) Independent sector *treatment centres*: how the NHS is left to pick up the pieces. *British Medical Journal 332*, p. 614.

Further reading

Ham, C. (2004) *Health Policy in Britain*, 5th ed. Basingstoke: Palgrave.

Peckham, S. and Exworthy, M. (2003) *Primary Care in the UK*. Basingstoke: Palgrave.

Sharkey, P. (2007) *The Essentials of Community Care*, 2nd ed. Basingstoke: Palgrave Macmillan.

Thomas, P. (2006) *Integrating Primary Health Care Leading, Managing, Facilitating*. Oxon: Radcliffe Publishing Ltd.

Watson, N. and Wilkinson, C. (2001) *Nursing in Primary Care*. Basingstoke: Palgrave.

Chapter 4

Outpatient nursing

Lioba Howatson-Jones

Learning objectives

(1) Identify the purpose and function of outpatient services
(2) Explore communication stances through critical reflection of personal value system
(3) Define the developing role of the nurse within outpatient services
(4) Consider health education and health promotion opportunities and influence on patient choice

---

Introduction

Definition

The outpatient department comprises clinic settings where referred patients consult with health professionals for diagnostic and monitoring purposes but are not admitted to hospital for that attendance.

Outpatient services in the United Kingdom (UK) have expanded dramatically in response to rising population need and health care advances. Since 1992 new attendances have increased by 4.7% annually and follow-up by 1.4% (Scott, 2000).

Seventy-two per cent of patients attending outpatients in 2000–2001 were doing so for follow-up and in 2001 284 000 patients were waiting >13 weeks for a first consultation (National Audit Office, 2001). Figures for 2001–2002 show a rise from 10.8 million attendances to 11.0 million. Included within these are new attendances which also rose from 3.1 to 3.2 million (Department of Health (DH), 2002). General and acute specialties account for 90% of this activity. Meeting this steady rise in demand requires thinking about service provision in different ways and considering the scope of professional roles has become the focus to expanding capacity. Until relatively recently, patients requiring the attention of a specialist were referred to a hospital-based setting. However, as elucidated in the previous chapter, health care reforms are moving services outside hospitals and closer to the patient's home in primary care. Specialty attendances, such as orthopaedics, general surgery, ophthalmology, dermatology, ear, nose and throat and gynaecology, traditionally provided by secondary care services in hospital, have been identified as suitable for provision in local primary care (DH, 2005). However, for some, referral to a hospital-based consultant may be more appropriate in order to encompass adjunct diagnostics reducing the number of attendances. The NHS Plan (DH, 2000) and Shifting the Balance of Power initiatives (DH, 2001a) establish a UK government commitment to listening to the views and needs of patients and involving them in decision making about their care. The work of outpatient clinics incorporates a wide range of conditions, specialties and patient population and is often the first contact that patients have with a specialist service. The encounter can leave a lasting impression influencing their attitude to health and disease management. Outpatient nursing, therefore, requires flexibility, a comprehensive knowledge base and the ability to engage with patients in a short space of time, helping them to make informed choices and decisions.

This chapter introduces two main areas. It firstly examines the function of outpatient services in providing specialist consultation, examination and treatment for patients who do not require acute inpatient admission. The purpose of consultation is differentiated between new and follow-up patient groups to demonstrate self-management strategies available to patients. Screening processes for selection of elective day service and inpatient admission are explained. Discharging patients from outpatient care and referring them on to other agencies is also considered in relation to the nature of activity of providing access to procedures, investigations or therapies.

Secondly, the chapter focuses on establishing a partnership between the patient and the nurse through issues of choice and communication, examining the role of the nurse. Patient expectations and concerns about the timing and structure of the clinic consultation and surrounding factors of equality, organisation, efficiency and accurate information are related to personal values and how these might influence viewing the local patient population and health promotion informing. Opportunities for the student to critically reflect on his/her own values and how these relate to becoming a critical practitioner in using different communication strategies and assessing written documentation are offered. The role of the nurse in health education, health promotion and advocacy through chaperoning is examined within national guidelines for education, training, safety and standards and role development (RCN, 2006). Opportunities for the student to make informed decisions about chaperoning are also explored.

Functions of outpatient services

Outpatient services provide non-acute ambulatory health care for a wide variety of conditions and through diverse forms, which include specialist and nurse-led clinics. Outreach services are also offered at sites closer to where patients live, such as health centres and general practitioner (GP) surgeries. These provide the same expertise as a *secondary-care* (hospital-sector)-based service. Most outpatient work is currently undertaken on a Monday-to-Friday basis usually in daytime hours with staff working flexi shifts. Units are extending their hours in recognition of the needs of those who have to work and to make more effective use of resources. Appointment slots are pre-booked, enabling patient choice to minimise disruption to their normal activity. Waiting times may vary, making it important for staff to keep patients informed of these on arrival. Teams that deliver outpatient services include receptionists (the first person the patient meets), medical staff (who often oversee and lead on patient management), nurses (who coordinate patient care and may take some case load), allied health professionals (AHPs) (who provide specific therapeutics), technicians (who undertake some investigations) and secretaries (who maintain the flow of information). All of these need to be aware of each other's roles and responsibilities and practise teamworking to facilitate smooth running of the service.

Cumulative knowledge

In what other centres might patients be able to access outpatient services?
(Refer back to Chapter 3 to check your answer.)

Nature of new activity

Patients with problematic symptoms will usually consult with their GP who may initiate some standard tests, such as blood tests. But, as primary care evolves, the practitioner they see may alternatively be a nurse, or AHP, as their roles develop and they take a greater lead in service provision and integrated care networks (Martin et al., 2007). Where required, onward referral to a specialist in that field enables patients to consult with, and gain treatment from, a practitioner who has specific expertise for their problem. The purpose of referral is for additional advice on diagnosis, treatment and access to further investigations not usually available in primary care (Clinical Standards Advisory Group (CSAG), 2000). The NHS Improvement Plan (2004) identified that waiting times were 17 weeks and demands that in future the patient's journey is completed within 18 weeks. These are much shorter for suspected cancer with a maximum wait of 2 weeks for suspected cancer referrals. The notes of new patients are reviewed before the clinic and a member of the team is assigned to see them. Where appropriate, patients may be directed to a one-stop clinic, which enables examination, investigation and early initiation of treatment in one setting. An example of this is a one-stop breast clinic where a patient who has found a lump is examined by a breast surgeon and undergoes

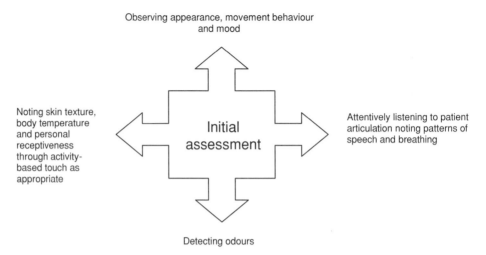

Figure 4.1   Assessment interaction.

mammography and possibly a breast biopsy. Being seen in this way enables early initiation of treatment by the surgeon.

Consultation

The purpose of consultation for new patients is to establish diagnosis, initiate suitable further investigations and exclude serious pathology (Gaunt, 2000). But such a narrow focus on condition limits opportunities for the patient participation envisaged by health care reform and challenges nurses to look more holistically at their activities with patients. On attending, patients are weighed and have baseline observations, such as pulse and blood pressure taken to assess current health status. This provides opportunity for assessment interaction and establishing a therapeutic relationship. Nurses use all their senses in completing assessment with patients in a very short period of time, as illustrated in Figure 4.1.

Tips & hints

Ask the patient how they feel today, why they are attending and what they would normally be doing. This enables them to give their own health assessment and clues to normal activity.

Patients are not familiar with the environment, or the staff, and may find it both intimidating and confusing. Staff need to introduce themselves and check how the patient wishes to be addressed. If it is necessary for patients to undress, they require a private area to do so with minimal external interference unless requesting help. To maintain privacy and dignity, consultations are conducted in a private area with only necessary staff present. Staff should avoid frequently going in and out of the room or leaving the patient alone in an isolated room for long periods, as this is unsettling. If intimate examination is necessary, a chaperone may be required (with patient consent). The specialist explains initial findings or interpretations of results and the intended course of action ensuring the patient understands and is agreeable before proceeding. Before leaving there is a further opportunity to engage the patient in participating in their own care by determining patient priorities and capabilities. If further specialist tests are necessary, patients need to have some idea of timescale, what is required of them and who to contact with enquiries.

Access to diagnostics and investigations

Most GP surgeries currently have limited diagnostic facilities, although they access a wider range of hospital-based services. A few are able to accommodate some services, but at present most need to refer patients to specialists who do have access and can directly act on the results. As technology advances, particularly in the field of telemedicine, research is being undertaken to identify the benefits of moving more diagnostics and a wider range of investigations further across the secondary and primary care interface to bring them closer to the patient (Martin et al., 2007). Other innovations include the picture archiving and communications system used in radiology settings, which stores images electronically enabling viewing from multiple sites by several professionals. Limitations are posed by the expense of investing in equipment and in maintaining specialist knowledge and competency. In future, a wider range of providers are likely to emerge, forming cooperatives to facilitate a service such as through, for example, a polyclinic, and private enterprise will provide entrepreneurial opportunities to professionals willing to branch out into business for themselves.

Screening for day or elective admission

Some diagnostic procedures need to be undertaken in a day setting where the patient may be admitted on a day-case basis, for example some endoscopy. Other indicative procedures may involve invasive techniques, for example some interventional radiological imaging or surgery requiring day surgery. Others may involve more extensive surgery, such as a hip replacement that, nevertheless, is not an acute emergency. A robust and in-depth assessment at the time of outpatient attendance helps to establish the right care environment for the patient and to make the best use of resources (DH, 2006a). Screening is based on:

- Intended procedure
- Patient medical history and diagnosis
- Investigation results
- Medication
- Current health status
- Ability to self-care and support network

For day surgery admission, this involves utilising the American Society of Anesthiologists (ASA) criteria, whilst for elective admission, a thorough anaesthetic assessment is necessary to identify suitability for surgery.

Cumulative knowledge

Which conditions exclude patients from day surgery admission according to the ASA criteria and why might this be? (See Chapter 6 on day surgery pre-assessment to find out more about the criteria.)

Leaving assessment to the time of admission may mean wasting patient and hospital time if they are found to be unsuitable. Pre-assessment is an increasing feature in determining suitability for many types of surgeries. Conversely, a number of minimally invasive surgical procedures are now carried out under local anaesthetic in the primary care setting avoiding hospital admission altogether, for example some hernia repairs.

Teaching and learning

Because of the diversity of the population and wide variety of conditions that patients present with, and the correspondingly broad knowledge base required, outpatient services provide good opportunities for training and learning for student and junior health professionals. When planning learning it is important to consider a realistic time frame, as well as to be sensitive to patient and carers needs and wishes. Where contact with learners is likely, advance warning is usually given and consent obtained from patients at attendance. Courtesy is observed by introducing learners and being sensitive regarding the content of teaching when the patient is present to avoid unduly alarming them (Royal College of Physicians, 2004). Nurses are in a position to expand the learning event to include aspects of holistic care and modes of communication in this short-term therapeutic environment, which promote sharing of skills and knowledge between professionals.

Nature of follow-up

Patients attend for follow-up after investigations for explanation of diagnoses and to determine ongoing care and management. Whilst patients know what to expect from having previously visited the clinic setting, they are still likely to be uncertain and worried about the outcome of the investigations they have undergone. The opportunity for personal interaction in seeing the patient face to face enables sharing information and participation in care planning.

Diagnosis of a chronic condition is not confined to the elderly but affects the young and middle aged as well, and these form the core of long-term attenders within outpatient services. Examples include individuals with conditions such as diabetes, heart disease, neurological and renal conditions amongst others.

Monitoring of chronic conditions involves accurate diagnosis and timely treatment to meet continuing and changing needs. This may also include rehabilitation and support services and the use of assistive technology, for example dialysis, and equipment to maximise patient potential and participation in an active life (DH, 2007). It relies on setting achievable goals that the patient can see the benefits of, and accurate patient reporting (Wellington, 2001). Follow-up, however, also seems to have continued a ritualistic pattern with some questioning its efficacy and necessity when initiated by the physician, as patient instigated follow-up results in fewer appointments and an increase in patient satisfaction (Hewlett et al., 2005).

It is envisaged that care planning will increasingly be managed in primary care through the introduction of community matrons working in advanced nursing roles that straddle the interface between hospital and community care, taking on some previously medically based strategies (Nursing and Midwifery Council (NMC), 2007a). The evidence base is still young and further research and development will help to mature this nursing role (Woodend, 2006). At the centre of managing chronic conditions is patient empowerment that facilitates informed choice and may have a role to play in reducing acute relapses and symptoms. Such facilitation of patient choice brings with it the realisation that some patients choose a different course not adherent with medical advice; such dilemmas require careful consideration (Metcalfe, 2005).

Health education versus health promotion

Health education imparts knowledge about specific health conditions, procedures and strategies giving the patient the information necessary to make informed choices about disease management and competing courses of action. As it is stimulated by a particular need, it is also guided by objectives related to fulfilling that need. In keeping with adult learning precepts, current knowledge should be assessed first to avoid diminishing patient self-concept and contribution. A variety of teaching modes may be used, such as verbal, written, visual and psychomotor, but those chosen are matched to the content and patient preference, or capability, and evaluated for effectiveness. Reinforcement may be required to renew understanding. The successfulness of the outcome is dependent on the degree to which health priorities fit in with the patient's belief system and capabilities, or indeed inclination, for fulfilment (Whitehead, 2004).

> **Reflection**
>
> What are your values in relation to health knowledge and behaviours and how might these influence your perception of patients?

Health promotion relates to activities that aim to enhance and support the well-being of the patient by focusing on perceptions of wellness and strategies that promote this and minimise, or prevent, ill health. An understanding of what an individual means by 'well-being' is central to the activities undertaken to promote and maintain it (Arnold, 2003). Traditional models of well-being have focused on the:

- Emotional
- Mental
- Social
- Spiritual
- Physical
- Environmental
  (Brenchley and Robinson, 2001, p. 1068)

But in seeking to empower individuals to change their own lives, they are also made accountable for their own health choices, which are impacted on by wider considerations, such as the 'environment, culture, economy and ecology' that are subject to political factors. Thus health also becomes a community endeavour (Whitehead, 2004). Health practitioners themselves are part of this community and role model aspects of health in their dealings with others and portrayal of themselves (Brenchley and Robinson, 2001). It is less likely that patients advised to modify a lifestyle choice will believe the benefits when the advisor is seen pursuing the same habit, for example smoking.

Checkpoint

The terms health education and health promotion are sometimes used interchangeably. How do they differ and where do they overlap?

Communication

The full range of communication strategies is employed to meet patient expectation and concern and facilitate efficient running of the clinic. Patient expectations include:

- Communication that is accurate and informative
- Fairness in administration of the clinic
- Organisation and efficiency
- Minimal waiting
- Friendly, informative and empathic staff
- Reasonable consultation time

The time of waiting for an appointment may create anxiety for patients and so clear written information is important to help orientation in what to expect, where to go for additional advice and where to report on the day of attendance. It is also important for patients to know what to do if they cannot make the appointment. These details are sent through preparatory correspondence with telephone numbers clearly displayed and any specific instructions such as bringing a list of medication or fasting for a blood test are included. Patients are asked to contact the department if they are hearing impaired or speak a different language requiring an interpreter. In some settings, nurses staff advice lines in order to give patients additional information. A wide variety of leaflets are also available, summarising diverse conditions in plain language and offering advice on how to manage effects and modify any contributing lifestyle issues. These are often written by patient groups. Consideration needs to be given to what patients are likely to be told at appointments and whether it would be beneficial for them to have someone with them (Royal College of Physicians, 2004).

Opportunity for the student

Using knowledge from reading about communication in Chapter 2 what different strategies might you employ in the running of a clinic to meet the patient expectations listed above and what is your reasoning for the choices you have made?

Written communication is a useful way of reinforcing information conveyed in other formats. It differs slightly from documentation in that its primary purpose is to communicate a message to the reader. Documentation on the other hand, while also fulfilling the role of communication, has the main purpose of providing a record of interactions with patients, and between professionals, as part of the professional requirement for documenting care given. It, therefore, includes all written forms, such as:

- Patient instructions
- Diagnostic requests and results
- Referral letters between health professionals
- Patient information letters
- Notes and patient records
- Care planning

Undermann Boggs and Langford (2003) recommend that written forms of communication are 'accurate, brief, complete and require specific professional writing skills' (p. 599). Table 4.1 summarises skills in relation to professional requirements of the NMC (2007b) for recorded documentation. Good written communication ensures dissemination of information within the multidisciplinary team promoting continuity of care between the diversity of departments and settings outpatients may visit, and fragmented episodes of attendance. It enhances the ability to detect any problems at an early stage. This helps to facilitate high standards of clinical care. It is also necessary to evidence health care processes by providing an accurate account of treatment, care planning and delivery.

Opportunity for the student

Examine the different types of written communication that are used within your particular outpatient service. How do they relate to the features and requirements described?

Table 4.1 Professional writing based on NMC (2007b) standards for record keeping

Content and style	Skills
Writing needs to include the facts and be consistent with these	Description and evaluation
Factual information should be recorded clearly and indelibly close to the event in consecutive order, including the date, time and signature of the writer for written records, or be attributable in electronic format. If alterations are required, these must be justifiable, dated and signed with the original entry still readable	Accuracy
Writing should not include abbreviations, jargon, irrelevant subjective or offensive statements and be written in a way that patients can understand	Clarity
Information on problems, risks and action taken as well as the care planned in association with patients and carers and information shared should be included	Summarising

The nurse's role

The nurse's role is pivotal in what is a busy and crowded arena for communicating, advocating and caring for the patient as appropriate. A conceptual view of the nurse's relationship to the patient and multidisciplinary team is offered in Figure 4.2.

Not all patients want to be involved in their own care, relying instead on the practitioner as expert. Advancing to person-centred care is context- and person dependent (Price, 2006). Policy also standardises care for specific conditions rather

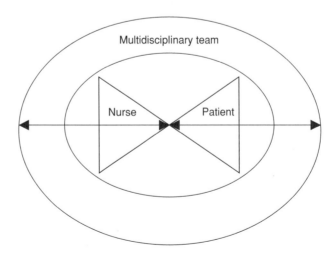

Figure 4.2 Conceptual view of the outpatient nurse's relationship to the patient and multidisciplinary team.

than individual patients. National Service Frameworks, for example, identify key interventions and strategies to be used. It is the nurses' role to mediate and interpret between the unique individual and the multidisciplinary team, assessing patient inclination and ability for self-determination. Although information may be passively received, providing opportunity for self-regulation interventions can empower patients and develop their coping strategies for disease management. Collaborative care includes patients and significant others. Being sensitive to advocacy opportunities, promoting evidence-based continuing care through professional working and maintaining a broad knowledge base through education and training to national guidelines is all part of the nursing role.

The Royal College of Nursing (RCN) (2006) has produced a detailed framework of specialist competencies for outpatient nurses identifying elements expected of differing levels of experience and expertise within the role. These include interacting with and supporting patients, using diverse specialist interventions, such as monitoring and multi-skilled interventions that assist with clinical procedures, preparation and problem solving, as well as discharge planning and health promotion. These are currently under review to reflect further developments in this diverse area of nursing.

Safety issues

Safety issues affect staff and patients alike. The environment of an outpatient service is busy and difficult to control. Patients expect to feel safe and secure and this may be achieved by orientating them to policies, physical layout and processes (DH, 2001b). Standards are addressed through the implementation of local policy, such as infection control, and national statute related to health and safety requirements. In particular, issues that may arise include:

- Exposure to hazards
- Manual handling
- Infection control
- Dealing with aggressive and violent behaviour
- Basic life support

It is part of the nurse's role to monitor for safety issues providing a prompt and knowledgeable response should these arise as part of minimising risk in accordance with the code of conduct (NMC, 2008). Where appropriate, patients also need to be made aware of their own responsibilities and actions in the fulfilment of safety procedures, for example manual handling. Decision making is directed towards addressing problems, delegating and reporting as required.

Opportunity for the student

Examine the local policies for the particular issues highlighted above. How might these relate to your role as a student?

Chaperoning

The intimate nature of health care procedures can expose both staff and patients to misinterpretation and accusation (RCN, 2002). Patients have a right to dignity and privacy that respects their personal boundaries, modesty, access to private changing facilities and independence (DH, 2001b). Nurses are accountable for promoting and protecting the interests of the patient (NMC, 2008) and in so doing are in a position to advocate for their needs within the multidisciplinary team. This requires sensitivity and assertiveness in identifying patient preference and requirement. Adopting a culture of openness and choice through full explanation and consent supports transparency of action and correct interpretation.

Research shows that those who have suffered adverse events such as rape or sexual abuse often need permission to disclose concerns, and this is dependent on the quality of the therapeutic relationships that are established with health personnel. It is part of the nurse's responsibility to advocate for this possibility. The recommended best practice for intimate procedures is to have a chaperone present as it provides protection for the patient and health care professional regardless of gender (Coldicott et al., 2003). Chaperones may include a friend or relative if the patient wishes but are more often the remit of the nurse. In all cases, where a chaperone is present, has been offered, but declined, or is unavailable, this should be documented in the notes (RCN, 2002). There may be occasions when an intimate examination may evoke a flashback to a previous adverse event. The person conducting the examination and the chaperoning nurse, if present, need to be sensitive to increasing anxiety and distress and stop the procedure immediately if requested to do so. A procedure should be allowed to continue only if the patient agrees and consents and termination of the procedure is documented in the notes.

Opportunity for the student

Discuss chaperoning examples with your mentor and the decision-making process in who fulfils the role and why.

Role development

Health care reform is focused on modernising nurses' roles and development around patient need (DH, 2006b). In particular, these are expected to fit into modern organisational models with diverse providers requiring greater flexibility and working across traditional boundaries. Establishing the evidence base for change and progression through research and audit helps to sustain embedding of developments, avoiding disintegration through lack of support. Areas of development include nurse-led care in multiple sclerosis, vascular, urology, pain, subfertility, dermatology, Macmillan services and many more. The future is likely to see an expansion of nurse-led provision venturing closer to the patients home and including many more minor operative interventions alongside consultation. As such, these roles could be said to be progressing in developing care alternatives, as opposed to a new role that still remains to be seen. Education and training play a key part in underpinning the expanding knowledge base required with many nurses now undertaking post-graduate studies.

Patient choice

Part of a commitment to delivering services closer to the patient includes providing choice to support accessibility and convenience for them (DH, 2006c). Patients now have the option of where they want to be seen and are able to make informed choices through publication of waiting times. As the electronic record project moves closer to completion, options for patient involvement increase through recording lifestyle choices and checking personal data online. Electronic booking is also moving closer to becoming available.

Referral and discharge

Regular reviewing of patient data and communication enables the identification of appropriate next steps. Sometimes referral to other members of the multidisciplinary team may be necessary, particularly if symptoms identify a different disease course or patient function alters requiring assistive services, for example if sight deficits prove to be neurological rather than ophthalmic in origin. The possibility of discharge may generate fear for some patients of being left to cope, and early preparation would help to alleviate some of these anxieties. Studies suggest that patients need clarity that discharge is going to occur and the reasons why it is happening in terms of cure, stability or simply wellness. Informing about disease and personal management are vital for patients not to feel abandoned and negative about the process (Burkey et al., 1997).

Scenario
Mrs Chacko is a 54-year-old, Hindu female, who speaks no English. She has been feeling very tired for some time and breathless on exertion. She has been referred by her general practitioner to the hospital for investigation of unexplained anaemia. She attends the outpatient department for an appointment with the consultant. She is accompanied by her husband who speaks good English. The consultant tells her husband that she needs a series of blood tests and a gastroscopy.

(1) What issues might the outpatient nurse want to consider in this scenario?
(2) What actions might she/he take?

Summary

Outpatient nursing has demonstrated an expanding field of operation and service provision. The nursing role is viewed in the context of supporting independent care decisions whilst taking an increasing lead in the provision of care. Opportunities for the student have been highlighted in applying communication knowledge within this short-term setting, examining features of written communication and documentation, exploring local policies and defining chaperoning decision making. Reflection on personal values in relation to health enables students to critically understand their responses to patient participation and health behaviours.

Acknowledgement

The author acknowledges the helpful discussions regarding nursing roles with Christine Cross, Clinical Sister, Outpatient Department, Medway Maritime Hospital.

Glossary of terms

Primary care
Service available in the community

Secondary care
Service available in an acute hospital

Websites

www.rcn.org.uk
www.dh.gov.uk

References

Arnold, E. (2003) Health promotion and client learning needs, in Arnold, E. and Boggs, K.U. (eds) *Interpersonal Relationships: Professional Communication Skills for Nurses*, 4th ed. St Louis, Missouri: Saunders, pp. 389–410.

Brenchley, T. and Robinson, S. (2001) Outpatient nurses, from handmaiden to autonomous practitioner. *British Journal of Nursing 10*(16), pp. 1067–1073.

Burkey, Y., Black, M. and Reeve, H. (1997) Patients' views on their discharge from follow up in outpatient clinics: qualitative study. *BMJ (Clinical Research Ed.) 315*(7116), pp. 1138–1141.

Clinical Standards Advisory Group (CSAG) (2000) *A Study of Hospital Outpatient Services Report of a CSAG Committee Chaired by Professor Pamela Enderby* [online]. Available from: http://www.dh.gov.uk/assetRoot/04/01/45/52/04014552.pdf (accessed 12 April 2007).

Coldicott, Y., Pope, C. and Roberts, C. (2003) The ethics of intimate examinations – teaching tomorrows doctors. *BMJ (Clinical Research Ed.) 326*, pp. 97–101.

Gaunt, M.E. (2000) *General Surgery Outpatient Decisions.* London: Arnold.

Department of Health (DH) (2000) *The NHS Plan.* London: HMSO.

Department of Health (2001a) *Shifting the Balance of Power Within the NHS: Securing Delivery* [online]. Available from: http://www.dh.gov.uk/assetRoot/04/07/65/22/04076522.pdf (accessed 19 July 2006).

Department of Health (2001b) *Essence of Care: Patient Focused Benchmarking for Health Care Practitioners.* London: HMSO.

Department of Health (2002) *Publication of Latest Statistics on Activity in Consultant Outpatient Clinics and A&E Departments, England, Quarter Ending 31 December 2001* [online]. Available from: http://www.dh.gov.uk/en/Publicationsandstatistics/Pressreleases/DH_4013060 (accessed 20 July 2007).

Department of Health (2004) *The NHS Improvement Plan.* London: HMSO.

Department of Health (2005) *Creating a Patient-Led NHS: Delivering the NHS Improvement Plan* [online]. Available from: http://www.dh.gov.uk/en/Publicationsandstatistics/Publications/PublicationsPolicyAndGuidance/DH_4106506 (accessed 11 April 2007).

Department of Health (2006a) *Reduce Wasted Bed Days, Improve Patient Care and Save Money – Hewitt.* Press release: 26th March 2006 [online]. Available from: http://www.dh.gov.uk/en/Publicationsandstatistics/Pressreleases/DH_4132360 (accessed 12 April 2007).

Department of Health (2006b) *Modernising Nursing Careers: Setting the Direction.* London: HMSO.

Department of Health (2006c) *Choice Matters: Increasing Choice Improves Patients' Experiences* [online]. Available from: http://www.dh.gov.uk/PublicationsAndStatistics/Publications/PublicationsPolicyAndGuidance/PublicationsPolicyAndGuidanceArticle/fs/en?CONTENT_ID=4135541&chk=Tcf9CM (accessed 19 July 2006).

Department of Health (2007) *The National Service Framework for Long-Term Conditions* [online]. Available from: http://www.dh.gov.uk/en/Publicationsandstatistics/Publications/PublicationsPolicyAndGuidance/Browsable/DH_4106042 (accessed 30 April 2007).

Hewlett, S., Kirwan, J., Pollock, J., Mitchell, K., Hehir, M., Blair, P.S., Memel, D. and Perry, M.G. (2005) Patient initiated follow up in rheumatoid arthritis: six year randomised control trial. *BMJ (Clinical Research Ed.) 330*, p. 171.

Martin, J., Black, G., Cleverdon, S. Kelly, D., Shanahan, H., Kinnair, D., Southon, S. and Webb, S. (2007) Developing service provision for patients in primary care. *Nursing Standard 21*(23), pp. 43–48.

Metcalfe, J. (2005) The management of patients with long-term conditions. *Nursing Standard 19*(45), pp. 53–60.

National Audit Office (2001) *Department of Health: Inpatient and Outpatient Waiting in the NHS.* London: National Audit Office.

Nursing and Midwifery Council (NMC) (2008) *The Code: Standards of Conduct, Performance and Ethics for Nurses and Midwives,* London: Nursing and Midwifery Council.

Nursing and Midwifery Council (2007a) *Advanced Nursing Practice – Update19 June 2007* [online]. Available from: http://www.nmc-uk.org/aArticle.aspx?ArticleID=2528 (accessed 20 June 2007).

Nursing and Midwifery Council (2007b) *Record Keeping* [online]. Available from: http://www.nmc-uk.org/aFrameDisplay.aspx?DocumentID=2699 (accessed 10 May 2007).

Price, B. (2006) Exploring person-centred care. *Nursing Standard 20*(50), pp. 49–56.

Royal College of Nursing (RCN) (2002) *Chaperoning: The Role of the Nurse and the Rights of Patients.* London: Royal College of Nursing.

Royal College of Nursing (2006) *Competencies: An Integrated Career and Competency Framework for Outpatient Nurses* [online]. Available from: http://www.rcn.org.uk/publications/pdf/outpatient_competency.pdf (accessed 19 July 2006).

Royal College of Physicians (2004) *How User Friendly Is Your Outpatient Department? A Guide for Improving Services.* London: Royal College of Physicians.

Scott, C. (2000) Clinical standards advisory group: services for outpatients. *Nursing Standard 14*(41), pp. 33–34.

Undermann Boggs, K. and Langford, D.R. (2003) Documentation in the age of computers, in Arnold, E. and Undermann Boggs, K. (eds) *Interpersonal Relationships: Professional Communication Skills for Nurses.* St Louis, Missouri: Saunders, pp. 573–606.

Wellington, M. (2001) Stanford health partners: rationale and early experiences in establishing physician group visits and chronic disease self-management workshops. *Journal of Ambulatory Care Management 24*(3), pp. 10–16.

Whitehead, D. (2004) Health promotion and health education: advancing the concepts. *Journal of Advanced Nursing 47*(3), pp. 311–320.

Woodend, K. (2006) The role of community matrons in supporting patients with long-term conditions. *Nursing Standard 20*(20), pp. 51–54.

Chapter 5

Minor injury and minor illness management

Roger Goldsmith and Karen Lumsden

Learning objectives

- Identify types and categories of presenting conditions
- Raise awareness of patient attendance issues and influences
- Consider communication strategies and their application to this setting
- Describe nursing roles and responsibilities

Introduction

Minor injury and minor illness (MIMI) management is a dynamic and significant part of emergency and primary care in the UK. Patients who use MIMI centres present with a variety of injury and illness pathologies and represent all section of society. The MIMI nurse must therefore be conversant with care for people from across the lifespan, from differing social and ethnic backgrounds and in various community settings.

Learners within the MIMI setting will have the opportunity to observe and, in some cases, participate in patient assessment, consultation and clinical examination, undertaking and ordering clinical investigations, diagnosis, delivering treatment and managing discharge and referral (e.g. to a general practitioner (GP) or to an orthopaedic team).

As part of the process of care delivery, learners will be able to experience how therapeutic communication is achieved despite the short-term nature of the MIMI setting and how patients' expectations may be met. Depending on the practice setting, it will be possible to observe the roles of a number of staff from within the inter-professional and support teams, including:

- Receptionists
- Registered nurses
- Nurse practitioners
- Doctors
- Health care assistants
- Allied health professionals (AHPs) (e.g. physiotherapists, occupational therapists and radiographers)

This chapter discusses the clinical settings in which MIMI care takes place, the rationale for patient attendance, understanding and delivering on patient expectations, the patient journey as well as principles of patient assessment and management. Nursing roles and responsibilities will also be explored in relation to risk assessment, informed consent, infection control, manual handling, health education and promotion.

Information about the patient journey is given together with patient expectations and detail of the clinical activity at each stage. Relevant communication issues are described for patients and for the health care team.

The clinical setting

Historically, minor injuries and minor illnesses were managed in either accident and emergency (A&E) departments or GP surgeries. The mid-1990s saw A&E departments gain a high profile as a result of the increasing patient numbers they were treating and the ensuing very long delays patients were experiencing when trying to access emergency care. Patients and the public raised concerns about the length of time they had to wait, even to be seen and treated for minor problems. As a result it was recognised that improvements in the management of 'walk-in' illness and injury treatment departments were needed.

Over the last few years the introduction of National Health Service (NHS) walk-in centres and minor injury units, which are often nurse led, community based and require no appointment, has helped improve access to emergency care. They are now an established and valuable part of local health care systems, providing care closer to patients' homes. NHS walk-in centres were established in 1999 to allow quick and easy access to a range of NHS services, including advice, information and treatment for a range of minor injuries and illnesses. Such reform and service redesign in relevant parts of the health care system, mainly primary care, meant that patients did not have to attend A&E departments.

In 2001, a 10-year strategy for 'reforming emergency care' was published to drive changes in emergency care and to give priority in terms of planning and resources to staff and patients in emergency care settings (Department of Health (DH), 2001a). The overarching aim of the strategy was to deliver services from the patient's perspective and offer high-quality, timely care for all patients wherever they access the system (Alberti, 2007).

Alongside the development of the new services for minor injuries and illnesses, clinical practice has also developed. An example of the development in clinical practice followed the review of emergency care services which led to the modernisation of service provision through the introduction of the 'See and Treat' initiative (DH, 2004a). The aim of this, essentially simple strategy, was to see patients immediately they walked in, assess their need for treatment and then provide it.

Although MIMI management now takes place in a variety of clinical settings, the care management goals and patient experience remain essentially the same in terms of short waiting times and good proximity to care providers.

Minor injury units

Minor injury units are designed to deal with minor injuries that happen like cuts and sprains. They may be located in small or large hospitals, attached to A&E departments or occasionally as stand-alone units. Minor injury units are typically nurse led and focused predominately on injuries but have developed, in some cases, to also manage minor illnesses. As with the traditional A&E no appointment is needed, but most minor injuries units do not treat patients under the age of 3.

Walk-in centres

NHS walk-in centres provide quick access to advice and treatment for minor injuries and illnesses (according to practitioner expertise and local protocol and guidelines), without an appointment. They have proved popular with the public with more than 4 million attendances between 2000 and 2004. They are designed to give patients more convenient access to a wider range of services. These centres are mainly nurse led but may have medical practitioners in residence as well. They may be located in stand-alone units in small, or large, hospitals and some are attached to A&E

departments. There are about 90 walk-in centres in the UK often open 7 days a week and some provide a 24 hour a day service.

Accident and emergency departments

A&E departments manage minor injury and minor illness in different ways; e.g. some continue to manage as they have traditionally done, while others have the MIMI management provided by nurse practitioners in a separate clinical area within them.

General practice surgeries and health centres

Minor illnesses can be treated in GP surgeries and health centres, as they always have been, by the GP themselves or by nurse practitioners. Some GP surgeries and health centres have developed a minor injury management provision for their registered patients.

Urgent treatment centres

Urgent treatment centres are becoming increasingly popular in a variety of locations as a means of supporting emergency and urgent care services within non-appointment primary care services. The model is in two main forms:

- A 'front door' pre-emergency department, located in an A&E department, where the service is a potential stream for patients attending without an appointment who have a minor injury or illness
- Remote services, in their own building, in some cases on existing community facilities such as a walk-in centre, minor injury unit or a community hospital

Some urgent treatment centres are also provided by the private sector.

Minor injury and minor illness

A minor injury is one that has occurred without a significant mechanism of injury or any significant trauma or sequelae. It is an injury that may require follow-up in terms of dressings and removal of sutures, but which can be managed appropriately within the resources of the setting and the expertise of the staff. An example of this would be a simple, uncomplicated finger dislocation which could be reduced with basic anaesthesia and pain relief.

- Common minor injuries include ankle sprains, minor head injuries, minor lacerations, radius and ulna fractures, foreign bodies within the eye, bruised ribs and minor abrasions.

> **Cumulative knowledge**
>
> Revise the physiology of bone healing.

A minor illness is an illness which is usually characterised by a sudden onset, e.g. an ear infection, although some can develop more insidiously, e.g. a fungal infection of the foot. The course of a minor illness is usually short, although some can present as chronic infections with relapse and remission.

Signs and symptoms, e.g. pain, are not so severe or significant that the patient cannot be discharged home with appropriate resources (e.g. advice, minor treatment or simple medication). Clinical investigations undertaken show at most only a minor deviation from normal values.

- Common minor illnesses include sore throats, earache, colds, coughs, minor chest infections, *epistaxis*, urinary tract infections, rashes and *conjunctivitis*.

> **Checkpoint**
>
> Consider the causes and effects of infection. What are the common signs and symptoms?

Roles and responsibilities

Within the MIMI setting the nursing staff have well-defined roles and responsibilities. Common roles and responsibilities of the nurse practitioner, registered nurse and health care assistant are highlighted in Table 5.1.

Table 5.1 Common roles and responsibilities of MIMI nursing staff

The nurse practitioner	*The registered nurse*
• Undertaking patient consultations • Diagnosing injury and illness • Prescribing treatments • Making decisions regarding patient discharge • Making appropriate referrals to other health care professionals	• Initial assessment and priority setting (e.g. triage) • Initial treatment (e.g. administering analgesia or undertaking wound dressings) • Giving support, explanation, information and advice • Carrying out or ordering investigations (e.g. urinalysis and X-rays) • Performing venepuncture • Undertaking further treatment procedures (e.g. suturing, applying plaster of Paris • Wound management

Health care assistant
Supports the trained nurses by undertaking clinical tasks and by giving support, explanation, information and advice to patients and significant others

The nurse practitioner

The nurse practitioner is a senior registered nurse who has expanded their role in the MIMI management setting. They carry out advanced nursing practice and manage the care of patients presenting with a minor injury or illness without direct medical supervision. They work collaboratively in partnership with other health care professionals making appropriate and timely referrals where necessary.

Reflection

What skills are needed by the nurse when making referrals to other health and social care professionals? How might these skills be developed?

Since 2004 the Nursing and Midwifery Council has undertaken a national consultation about the status of nurses who hold job titles that imply an advanced level of knowledge and competence and who often work independently. In 2005, the council agreed that 'advanced nurse practitioner' should be a registerable qualification and is seeking approval from government for opening a further 'subpart' to the nurses' part of the register (Nursing and Midwifery Council (NMC), 2007).

Nurse practitioners demonstrate an appropriate knowledge of applied anatomy, physiology and pathophysiology relevant to patients with a minor injury or illness and they can undertake effective assessments and examinations of patients and following this decide on any investigations required. Nurse practitioners are able to set appropriate priorities and make beneficial decisions regarding the management of a patient's care and reflect critically on the treatment of the patient, management of his/her pathology and the effectiveness of the strategies adopted. They constantly evaluate the knowledge and skills required to work effectively within the collaborative practice model of patient care. Typically the nurse practitioner has undertaken an advanced-level training within the higher education setting.

Nursing responsibilities

Nurses have responsibility for effective care management at every stage of the patient's journey through the MIMI care setting. As well as the clinical focus of their work they ensure that patients' dignity, privacy and confidentiality are maintained and that informed consent is obtained (NMC, 2008). In common with all other health and social care professionals nurses within the MIMI setting are required to ensure that all patients are treated equally irrespective of race, gender, age, social and economic background, sexual orientation or cause of their injury or illness (Social Care Institute for Excellence, 2007).

Reflection

Reflect on the key ethical principles. Consider which ones apply to the goals outlined above.

Box 5.1 Examples of clinical tasks undertaken in MIMI centres

Wound cleaning and dressing
Applying Plaster of Paris back slabs
Venepuncture
Obtaining an electrocardiogram
Monitoring vital signs
Simple wound closure (e.g. using wound glue)
Assisting with suturing
Applying splints and slings

The roles of the nurse working within the MIMI environment are many and varied, and staff there need to have a broad knowledge and practical skill base to deal with the wide range of problems which patient present with. Box 5.1 gives some examples of the clinical tasks that nurses undertake in the MIMI centre. As well as the more specialist tasks, the nurse is also responsible for ensuring that patients' expectation of high standards in respect of general issues, such as infection control and manual handling, are fully met.

Clinical procedures

The nurse practitioner's clinical practice is usually informed by protocols that indicate what minor injury and minor illness pathologies they can, and cannot, treat. Within the protocols there is information and direction on decisions to be made, treatments to be prescribed and the choice of discharge or referral pathways appropriate to a given condition. This is often achieved through the use of flow charts and treatment algorithms. There are strategies in place for the ongoing support, guidance and professional development of the nurse practitioner, e.g. via senior doctors within an A&E department or more formally through education and training, within both the hospital and university settings.

Infection control and manual handling

Given the high numbers and rapid turnover of patients treated in the emergency care setting, effective manual handling and infection control are of particular importance (review Chapter 7 on radiological procedures for guidance in these two areas). As with all areas in which health care takes place the key tenets of universal precautions need to be adhered to at all times. This means that the nurses in the MIMI centre will treat all patients as if they are potentially infectious, thereby safeguarding themselves, their colleagues and other patients.

The high turnover of patients through the department means that there is an ever-present temptation to cut corners to get the job done quickly. In common with all health care settings, however, nurses have a responsibility to themselves and to others to ensure that their practice is safe and that they observe the usual moving and handling conventions.

> **Opportunity for the student**
>
> Think about your manual handling training and discuss with staff how they manage the manual handling of patients within the minor injuries and illness setting. Discover what aids and devices for manual handling are available and how they are used.

Patient attendance

Patient patterns of attending a MIMI setting vary widely and reflect such influences as:

- The geographical setting
- The social, economic and ethnic makeup of the community it serves
- Local business, tourist and visitor activity
- The work profile of its inhabitants and their leisure pursuits
- The traffic volumes and travel options
- The age and gender mix of the community

A great majority of patients with minor illnesses and minor injuries self-refer, although some are advised, or directed, to attend by other health care professionals, e.g. GPs, ambulance service and NHS direct personnel. Most patients arrive using their own transport, although occasionally patients with a minor injury and minor illness may arrive by ambulance or accompanied by police officers.

Minor illnesses may have been present for some days, or the patient may attend as soon as they are aware of a problem. Similarly patients may attend as soon after the injury as possible or may have waited a varying amount of time from hours to days or occasionally weeks before seeking help or advice. Significant numbers of patients have tried remedies and treatments of their own choosing prior to attendance and some have been seen and treated initially by other health care professionals before deciding or being advised to attend. A small proportion of patients reattend because their symptoms are not improving.

Part of the role of the nurse practising within the MIMI environment is to ascertain through careful questioning the history of the problem. An understanding of the background of the patient, the history of the illness or injury and the reasons for the timing and mode of presentation to the centre may give vital clues as to the cause of the illness or injury and the patient's understanding of its management. Strategies for communication are discussed in detail in Chapter 2.

> **Opportunity for the student**
>
> Find out the history of a minor illness/injury of a patient you meet. Find out why they have attended at the time they have and why they have chosen to attend the particular unit they have.

Some years ago, if a patient was deemed by health care professionals to have failed to use the service properly then they could be labelled an 'inappropriate attender' (Purcell, 2003). This label is now itself deemed 'inappropriate'. Practitioners have a duty of care for any patient seeking advice or treatment.

In MIMI settings practitioners are skilled at assessing any patient and responding in the most appropriate way. This may be treating the patient at the unit, directing them to a more appropriate health care professional (e.g their GP or the emergency dental service) or giving advice about pharmacy and physiotherapy services, for example. Such attendances are a common occurrence with patients seeking advice and treatment for a whole range of pathologies that they, the patient, cannot be expected to either self-treat or work out where they might be most appropriately treated. It is necessary that the staff in the MIMI centre remember that the range of options for treatment may themselves lead to confusion for members of the public and that understanding the causes and treatments for minor ailments is something that most members of the public are not trained to do.

Attribution theory

Attribution theory is a theory in social psychology developed by Fritz Heider in the 1950s. The theory is concerned with the ways in which people explain, or attribute, the behaviour of others, or themselves (self-attribution), to something else. It investigates how individual's 'attribute' causes to outcomes and how this perception affects how they feel about things.

The theory divides the way people attribute causes to events into two types:

- External or situational
- Internal or dispositional
  (Heider, 1958)

External, or situational, attribution assigns causality to outside factors, like the seasons, leisure activities, type of work practices or availability of health care provision at a certain time.

Internal, or dispositional, attribution assigns causality to factors within the person, such as their level of intelligence or other variables, which make the individual responsible for the event such a propensity to drink alcohol to excess, take risks or their ability to make decisions and choices regarding their personal health.

Personality type may, therefore, impact on the timing of, reasons for and manner of attendance of the individual patient. The nurse should be accepting of the fact that some people are unable to make the best choices about their own care and that they will attend the most convenient, not necessarily the most appropriate, facility.

Attributional type may also affect an individual's ability to cooperate with treatment regimens; this should be accounted for in the decisions the nurse makes at the point of care. As such personality types will also have an impact on the plans for discharge and follow-up requiring that the nurse has considered the appropriateness of the decisions they make.

Reflection

Think about how an understanding of attribution theory might assist a nurse in understanding and treating a patient's condition in this setting. Could an understanding of attribution theory impact on the nurse's perception of the patient?

The patient journey

This section seeks to examine distinct areas of the patient journey, identifying what happens, when, who is responsible and the potential to affect the patient experience of care (Table 5.2).

- Booking in: Initial contact is usually with a receptionist who registers the attendance and the nature of the presenting problem and creates patient documentation, including demographic data, for use by the clinical staff.
- Initial assessment: The person undertaking the initial clinical assessment will assess patient need, priority of intervention and consideration of whether the clinical setting is the most appropriate one for the patient. The assessing practitioner, or nurse, interviews the patient, discovers their reason for attending, explains the

Table 5.2 A schematic of the patient journey through a MIMI centre

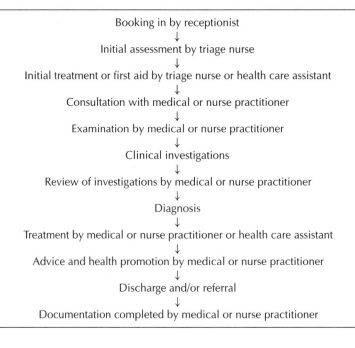

Booking in by receptionist
↓
Initial assessment by triage nurse
↓
Initial treatment or first aid by triage nurse or health care assistant
↓
Consultation with medical or nurse practitioner
↓
Examination by medical or nurse practitioner
↓
Clinical investigations
↓
Review of investigations by medical or nurse practitioner
↓
Diagnosis
↓
Treatment by medical or nurse practitioner or health care assistant
↓
Advice and health promotion by medical or nurse practitioner
↓
Discharge and/or referral
↓
Documentation completed by medical or nurse practitioner

role and resources of the unit and outlines what the patient can expect from the episode of care. Any appropriate clinical observations (e.g. blood pressure and temperature) are taken at this time. Triage, using a formal framework to inform assessment of need and the setting of priorities for care management, is one method of structuring this process.

- Initial treatment or intervention: This is an intermediate step taken to make the patient more comfortable prior to a more formal and thorough examination. At this stage the patient may be supplied with analgesia, a wound dressings or a wheelchair for example.
- Consultation/taking a history: A comprehensive discussion and interview with the patient is an integral part of a patient assessment. The most important task of the consultation is to make a diagnosis: this is crucial for determining the patient's presenting problem and deciding on their subsequent treatment. In addition to comprehending the physical nature of the presenting problem, an understanding of the psychological and social aspects of the problem is also vital for making a successful diagnosis.

There are a number of models that the nurse practitioner may use to structure their communication with the patient at this stage of their care management. An example of this is Neighbour's *The Inner Consultation* model, which sets curiosity as a central theme in patient-centred consultation (Neighbour, 1987) and is given in Box 5.2.

There are other models which some practitioners may find more appropriate to their practice. Readers are referred to other models such as those by Pendelton et al. (1984) and Byrne and Long (1976), which, despite their age, remain seminal works still informing consultations in practice.

Box 5.2 Neighbour's inner consultation model (1987)

Neighbour's five checkpoints in the consultation:

(1) *Connecting*: Have the practitioner and the patient got a rapport?

(2) *Summarising*: Can the practitioner demonstrate to the patient that they have sufficiently understood why he or she has come:

What is the patient's reason for attending?

What are the patient's ideas and feelings? Concerns and expectations are explored at this stage and acknowledged.

The practitioner listens and elicits patient responses.

The practitioner undertakes the clinical process of assessment, diagnosis, explanation, negotiation and agreement with the patient.

(3) *Handing over*: Has the patient accepted the agreed management plan?

(4) *Safety netting*: What if problems or complications occur? The practitioner:

Predicts what could happen if things go well?

Discusses how to manage an unexpected turn of events.

Considers plans and contingency plans.

(5) *Housekeeping*: Is the practitioner in a good condition for the next patient? Is there any stress and are they able to concentrate and maintain equanimity?

Box 5.3 A model elbow examination

> *Inspection and palpation*: The patient's forearm is supported with the opposite hand, so the elbow is flexed to 70°. The medial and lateral epicondyles and the olecranon process of the ulna are identified. The contours of the elbow including the extensor surface of the ulna and the olecranon process are inspected; any nodules and swelling are noted.
>
> The olecranon process and the epicondyles are palpated for tenderness; any displacement of the olecranon is noted. The grooves between the epicondyles and the olecranon are palpated, noting any tenderness, swelling or thickening.
>
> *Range of motion and manoeuvres*: Range of motion includes flexion and extension at the elbow and pronation and supination of the forearm. In order to test flexion and extension the patient is asked to bend and straighten the elbow. With the patient's arms at the sides and elbows flexed to minimise shoulder movement the patient is then asked to supinate, or turn up the palms, and to pronate, or turn the palms down (Bickley, 2007).

Clinical examination

The practitioner's clinical examination of a patient is a skilled and organised activity, undertaken with care and consideration and with the consent of the patient. It may be necessary at this stage to seek the verbal consent of the patient to examine them and in some cases the attendance of a chaperone is advisable.

Two examples of common clinical examinations are given below one from a of minor injury and the other from a minor illness scenario.

Minor injury

Elbow injuries, often the result of a fall, are common presentations to minor injury units. An outline of an elbow examination is given in Box 5.3.

> **Reflection**
>
> Review the anatomy and physiology of the elbow. Can you name the bones, muscle groups and additional structures of the elbow? Are you able to describe the normal range of movements at the elbow?

Minor illness

Earache is a common condition presenting to MIMI settings. An outline of an ear examination is given in Box 5.4.

> **Reflection**
>
> Review your knowledge of the anatomy and physiology of the ear. Can you describe the anatomy of the outer and inner ear and recall the physiology of hearing?

Box 5.4 A model ear examination

> *The auricle*: Each auricle and surrounding tissues are inspected for deformities, lumps or skin lesions.
>
> *Ear canal and drum*: An otoscope is used to inspect the ear canal: any discharge, foreign bodies, redness of the skin or swelling are noted. The ear drum is inspected and its colour and contour are noted.
>
> *Auditory acuity*: An estimation of hearing, testing one ear at a time.
>
> *Air and bone conduction*: If hearing is diminished, an assessment is made to see if the loss is conductive or sensoneural (Bickley, 2007).

Investigations and review of investigations

The role of investigations is to obtain and review clinical data in order to assist the practitioner in reaching a diagnosis. Examples of simple clinical investigations include urinalysis, blood tests and X-rays.

After the initial consultation with the patient during which the history and symptoms of the presenting problem are ascertained, the nurse practitioner establishes a working definition of the problem, made at the highest level of explicitness and certainty that the data allow (Bickley, 2007).

To make a diagnosis, or solve a problem, it is necessary to generate an appropriate working diagnosis or identify problems according to circumstances by seeking relevant and discriminating physical signs to help confirm, or refute, the working diagnosis. This involves interpreting and correctly applying information obtained from patient records, history, examination and investigations. This information is then interpreted using the nurse's knowledge of the basic, behavioural and clinical sciences to assist in the identification, management and resolution of the patient's problems. Throughout the process the nurse has to recognise the limits his/her own competence, act appropriately and seek further assistance if required (Fraser, 1992).

Treatments

Once a diagnosis has been established and a plan of care drawn up, the nurse working in the MIMI centre will initiate treatment; this may mean undertaking the task themselves, delegating the task to a colleague or referring the patient on. Some of the common treatments and aids provided in minor injury management include the undertaking, provision or application of:

- Slings
- Arthropads
- Splints
- Sutures
- Steristrips
- Elastoplast

- Wound glue
- Simple analgesia
- Plaster of Paris casts
- Trephining
- Crutches
- Dressings
- Wound cleansing

Whilst some of the common procedures in minor illness management include:

- Cleaning and dressing of infected areas
- Incision and drainage of minor abscesses
- Provision and administration of oral or topical medication such as antibiotics
- Provision and administration of other medication such as bronchodilators, simple analgesia and anti-inflammatories or simple laxatives

Health education and health promotion

As well as managing the presenting problem, staff in the MIMI setting undertake many health education and health promotion activities. Although these activities are often, from necessity, brief due to the numbers of patients and the short-term nature of their attendance, the importance of health education and promotion is not underestimated. It may be that the education applies to the presenting condition, a lifestyle choice or behaviour and that the intervention of the nurse at this stage allows the patient to make some more informed choices about their condition or their lifestyle.

Health promotion and educational activities are not restricted to the consulting room; examples of such activity may be observed in many areas of the clinical setting and include:

- Posters
- Leaflets
- Advice cards
- Verbal advice
- Immunisation and vaccination
- Communication on notifiable diseases notifications
- Referral to specialist practitioners such as physiotherapists, dentists and sexual health practitioners

Managing discharge

Given that it is intended that a great many patients will attend a minor injury/illness setting only once for any given complaint, it is vital that their discharge is managed effectively and safely. A majority of patients are discharged home with no specific follow-up, although in these circumstances advice is always given regarding reattendance, or attendance elsewhere, if problems recur or if the patient has any further worries or concerns.

Any possible complication, and the expected progression of the injury or illness, is explained, along with any instruction and advice needed regarding treatment undertaken, or prescribed, in the unit both to the patient and significant others (where appropriate). Some patients are referred to follow up outpatient department clinics, such as fracture or ophthalmology clinics, for continuing management or review. Some patients are referred to their GP for further management and interventions like the redressing of wounds, whilst others are referred on to specialist clinics. Many units also have their own 'in-house' review clinics run by nurse practitioners or senior medical staff.

Plans for discharge are started from the moment of attendance to the MIMI centre and are refined during the patient–practitioner consultation. The importance of good-quality communication and understanding of the patient's home circumstances are fundamental.

Referral and transfer

Clinical settings in which minor injuries and illnesses are seen manage those injury and illness pathologies that they cannot themselves treat by referring them on (and if needed arranging transfer), to appropriate clinical settings, e.g. to a paediatric unit or an A&E department. Staff must ensure that the referral is effective and that any transfer is safely facilitated using the most appropriate means; on occasion this may mean an ambulance being used with an accompanying nurse escort.

Documentation

Accurate, comprehensive documentation of a patient episode is vital for ensuring that patients receive effective continuation of their care and that all details of the episode are available to those individuals authorised to have access to it. Poor, or missing, documentation may result in inefficient, or ineffective, care being given during the minor injury and minor illness care episode or by agencies to whom the patient is later referred.

Documentation may be handwritten or computerised, or both. Apart from clinical notes (see Box 5.5), evidence of time spent in the unit, time between clinical actions for example, may be collated and documented and is often known as 'patient tracking'. Such tracking serves to prove that the unit has met the local and national targets for waiting and treatment times (no longer than 4 hours since 2004) as well as providing valuable insights into the nature and numbers of illnesses and injuries seen within the unit. Such data may be used to plan the locations and resourcing of future units and the MIMI unit itself. Documentation also provides evidence for auditing the ability of the centre to meet benchmarks such as 'promoting health' in the essence of care initiative (DH, 2006), National Service Frameworks – for example 'older people' (DH, 2001b) and 'children' (DH, 2004b).

Box 5.5 Examples of standard abbreviations used in clinical notes

Presenting complaint (pc) – the reason why the patient is seeking help from a medical or nurse practitioner

History of presenting complaint (hpc) – a chronological record of the complaint
Past medical history (pmh) – significant/relevant injury or illness
Drug history (dh) – current medication; also known allergies
Family history (fh) – information related to hereditary illnesses
Social history (sh) – important (personal) information relating to the social and work situation of the patient

Functional enquiry (if required) – systematic record of the functioning of organ systems not covered in the history of presenting complaint

On examination (o/e) – positive and negative findings from clinical examination
Impression (imp) – provisional diagnosis/es
Plan – investigations, tests, interventions, treatments to be undertaken
Findings/results – from investigations/tests
Diagnosis
Prescription – to include treatments/follow-up/advice etc.

Other examples of documentation which are created within the MIMI unit are letters to GPs, giving details of patient injury or illness and their management and the generation of outpatient department appointments. Any untoward incidents (e.g. patient complaints, difficult behaviour or accidents in the unit) are also to be documented.

Clinical notes

The notes that a nurse practitioner writes will conform to a locally agreed structure. This means that other professionals subsequently accessing the notes know what to look for and where and when they need answers to important clinical questions. It is also important in demonstrating that the care given to a patient has actually taken place and is invaluable in this respect in a court of law. It is usual within the clinical notes to see the use of standard abbreviations. Examples of standard abbreviations are given in Box 5.5.

Opportunity for the student

Observe how individualised person-centred care is achieved at each stage of the patient journey.

Communication with the patient

Some aspects of this communication have been dealt with earlier when considering the patient's initial assessment, consultation and health promotional and educational activities with the MIMI unit. The health care team in the clinical setting all endeavour to communicate effectively and therapeutically with patients, and their significant others, regardless of the mode or reason for presentation, whilst taking into consideration issues of patient age, gender, ethnicity and social and cultural needs. Patients present with many different behaviours and emotions; they are often distressed and often in varying degrees of pain. Some attenders are under the influence of alcohol and drugs and may prove difficult to communicate with.

A number of strategies may be used to aid communication; these include:

- Verbal: e.g. explanation, advice and reassurance
- Visual: e.g. pictures and the internet resources
- Non-verbal: e.g. touch, eye contact and maintaining an appropriate interpersonal distance
- Printed: e.g. advice cards and leaflets

Reflection

How might you apply your knowledge of communication theory to distressed patients in pain? What communication strategies are used in the MIMI setting which address issues of patient age, ethnic background and presenting complaint?

Observation of a strict code of obtaining informed consent from patients within the MIMI setting prior to history taking, examination, investigations, treatments, referral, follow-up and discharge will both contribute to a high quality of care provision and improve the patient experience. Obtaining consent can present some challenges for the nurse practitioner due to the diversity of patients attending the MIMI unit and the ephemeral nature of the relationship. For the principles of informed consent, see Chapter 2 on communication and ethics.

Reflection

Reflect on the principles of informed consent. Given the short-term nature of MIMI management how might you ensure that that it is obtained in a manner which reflects these principles?

Effective communication within the health care team in a unit and between that team and other health care professionals, outside agencies and other clinical settings is vital for optimal patient care. The important role of documentation in aiding communication has already been discussed in this chapter. Communication is particularly important in special circumstances where, for example, non-accidental injury or elder abuse is suspected.

There are a significant number of individuals to consider; e.g. nurse practitioners may need to communicate with:

- Doctors
- Other nurse practitioners
- A&E, paediatric, community and mental health nurses
- Ambulance personnel
- Radiographers

- Porters
- Biochemists
- Police
- Nurse managers
- Cleaners
- Receptionists
- Physiotherapists

Communication may be:

- Verbal: face to face or telephone
- Via e-mail
- Written/computer generated: e.g. letters and patient notes
- Images sent via the internet: e.g. photographs of wounds
- The scrutiny of X-ray images and results of investigations which can be visualised and discussed hospitalwide via computer links
- Trust intranet

Opportunity for the student

Observe the communication pathways available, for example, for contacting on-call doctor services, out-of-hour social services or transport services.

Scenario

Minor injury

Mr Brunt is a 70-years-old retired solicitor. He developed a persistent tremor in his hands and was finding walking a problem prior to being diagnosed with Parkinson's disease last year. Mr Brunt lives with his elderly partner in a semi-detached house. He attends the minor injury unit having injured his arm in a fall earlier today. He has a superficial wound on his elbow that is swollen and bleeding. Mr Brunt is anxious and upset and indicates that he needs to get home as soon as possible.

(1) How will this patient be managed in the minor injury unit?
(2) What issues in terms of communication, dignity and team working are likely to arise?

Minor illness

Ms Drobkov is 23 years old. She originates from Slovakia and speaks little English. She currently works as a fruit packer and is not registered with a GP. She has enjoyed good health up to now. She presents to the minor injury and illness unit complaining of feeling unwell. A friend, and co-worker, says she can help with translation.

The triage nurse establishes that Ms Drobkov has frequency of urine, burning on micturition, lower abdominal pain and feels hot.

What investigations should be undertaken and what might they show?
What ethical issues might arise?
What are relevant issues for continuing care planning?

> **Reflection**
>
> Considering both the scenarios, how does a minor injury and its management differ from that of a minor illness?

Summary

Minor injury and minor illness nursing has been demonstrated as taking place within a changing, dynamic and challenging arena with significant patient expectation. The nursing role has been considered in the context of a multidisciplinary team requiring effective communication and management skills. Opportunities for the student have been highlighted for communication pathways, patient attendance, individualised person-centred care and manual handling, together with reflection on ethical principles and clinical practice.

Glossary of terms

Conjunctivitis
Conjunctivitis is an inflammation of the conjunctiva most commonly due to an allergic reaction or an infection (usually bacterial or viral)

Epistaxis
An epistaxis is the relatively common occurrence of haemorrhage from the nose, usually noticed when it drains out through the nostrils. The common name for epistaxis is a 'nosebleed'

Otoscope
An otoscope or auriscope is a medical device which is used to look into the ears. With an otoscope, it is possible to visualise the outer ear and middle ear. Otoscopes consist of a handle and a head. The head contains an electric light source and a low-power magnifying lens. The front end of the otoscope has an attachment for disposable plastic ear speculums

Palpation
Palpation is used as part of a physical examination in which an object is felt to determine its size, shape, firmness or location

Trephining
A form of surgery in which a hole is drilled into a finger, or toe, nail to release the pressure of a haematoma that has formed between the nail and the nail bed below it

Websites

www.doh.gov.uk
www.gpnotebook.co.uk
www.nice.org.uk
www.nmc-uk.org
www.rcn.org.uk

References

Alberti, G. (2007) *Emergency Care Ten Years on: Reforming Emergency Care*. London: HMSO.

Bickley, L.S. (2007) *Bates' Guide to Physical Examination and History Taking*, 9th ed. Philadelphia: Lippincott Williams and Wilkins.

Byrne, P.S. and Long, B.E.L. (1976) *Doctors Talking to Patients*. London: HMSO.

Department of Health (DH) (2001a) *Reforming Emergency Care: first steps to a new approach*. London: HMSO.

Department of Health (DH) (2001b) *National Service Framework for Older People*. London: HMSO.

Department of Health (DH) (2004a) *Making See and Treat Work for Patients and Staff*. London: HMSO.

Department of Health (DH) (2004b) *National Service Framework for Children*. London: HMSO.

Department of Health (DH) (2006) *Essence of Care: Promoting Health*. London: HMSO.

Fraser, R.C. (1992) *Clinical Method: A General Practice Approach*, 2nd ed. London: Butterworth Heinemann.

Heider, F. (1958) *The Psychology of Interpersonal Relations*. New York: John Wiley & Sons.

Neighbour, R. (1987) *The Inner Consultation*. Lancaster: MTO Press.

Nursing and Midwifery Council (2008) The *Code: Standards for Conduct, Performance and Ethics for Nurses and Midwives*. London: Nursing and Midwifery Council.

Nursing and Midwifery Council (NMC) (2007) *Advanced Nursing Practice – Update 19 June 2007* [online]. Available from: http://www.nmc-uk.org/aArticle.aspx?ArticleID=2528 (accessed 20 June 2007).

Pendelton, D. Schofield, T. Tate, P. and Havelock, P. (1984) *The Consultation: An Approach to Learning and Teaching*. Oxford: Oxford University Press.

Purcell, D. (2003) *Minor Injuries: A Clinical Guide*. Edinburgh: Churchill Livingstone.

Social Care Institute for Excellence (2007) *Practice Guide 09: Dignity in Care* [online]. Available from: http://www.scie.org.uk/publications/practiceguides/practiceguide09/index.asp (accessed 2 October 2007).

Chapter 6

Preoperative assessment in day surgery

Beverley McNeil

Learning objectives

After reading this chapter and participating in the activities, the reader should have a clearer understanding of:

- Why and how effective preoperative assessment can lead to greater efficiency and reduce cancellations
- The skills necessary for effective preoperative assessment of patients
- The type of questions asked at preoperative assessment
- How patients are deemed, suitable or unsuitable, for day surgery
- Some of the basic investigations instigated by the preoperative assessment practitioner
- The type of information routinely given to patients

Introduction

Definition

Preoperative assessment is the process by which an individual's suitability for day surgery is determined. The pre-assessment practitioner must ensure that the individual scheduled for day surgery has a full understanding of the procedure to be undertaken, and wishes to proceed. During pre-assessment, the patient's past medical history is investigated and examination of baseline parameters is undertaken (usually pulse and blood pressure, although physical examination may occasionally be necessary). The findings establish patient fitness for both surgery and anaesthesia, which in turn determines their suitability for receiving treatment within a day surgery unit. Of equal importance, the pre-assessment process should identify the need for any specific instruments or equipment over and above normal resources. Discharge arrangements and the patient's home support are also discussed.

The early 1990s saw considerable expansion in the use of day surgery with establishment of many new facilities. By the end of the decade however, the initial rise in patient throughput levelled off, and a decline in productivity was witnessed within some day surgery units. At the same time there was recognition of the need to raise capacity within the National Health Service (NHS) in order to meet increasing demand, and day surgery was seen as an important means by which this could be achieved. The NHS plan acknowledged the potential for day surgery to make an important contribution towards helping the NHS achieve its target of treating more patients more promptly and proposed that 75% of elective surgery should be undertaken on a day case basis (Department of Health (DH), 2000).

Worryingly, an audit commission report, released in 2001, revealed that day surgery units were generally *not* performing at maximum capacity levels. If all units conformed to the standards of the most efficient, it was estimated there would be the potential to undertake an additional 120 000 operations each year. Hence, in 2002, the day surgery strategy was launched with the aim of promoting day surgery provision within the NHS. This was facilitated by the enthusiasm and assistance of the British Association of Day Surgery (BADS), a multidisciplinary council established in 1989 with the aim of progressing day surgery (DH, 2000, 2002a; McMillan, 2005).

In 2002, £68 million was made available for improvements to the efficiency and effectiveness of the NHS, in particular, to address the problem of 'blockages' causing cancellations and delays. In addition to speeding up progress with day case bookings, funding was made available for additional medical equipment and small building work for those organisations without separate day case facilities (DH, 2002a). It was established that day surgery is most successful when undertaken within a purpose-built unit, or one which has been converted for day surgery purposes, deliberately remote from the main operating theatre suite. There are many reasons for this; primarily, where day surgery is undertaken within a main theatre complex, patient cancellations may follow the arrival of unexpected emergency or trauma patients, who naturally take precedence over elective cases. Moreover, operating lists composed of both inpatients and day cases have historically resulted in day case cancellations when operating time expired, since surgeons preferred to deal with longer, more complicated cases at the beginning of the list and were not averse to delegating minor cases to slower, more junior staff (DH, 2002a).

Additionally, utilisation of inpatient operating theatres and inpatient wards for day surgery is not recommended, since same-day discharge is less successful, with 'stay-in' rates rising from 2.4% within stand-alone units to 14% where inpatient facilities are used (DH, 2002a). Hence, working within a self-contained, purpose-built unit is seen to lead to greater efficiency with operating time ring-fenced and all the services to hand. Where mixed lists in main operating theatre suites must occur, day surgery cases should be scheduled early on the list to prevent cancellations and allow adequate time for recovery before discharge (DH, 2002a).

Along with the extra funding, a new *Day Surgery: Operational Guide* was published, with the purpose of assisting managers and clinicians to improve day surgery rates through reduction in waiting times, introduction of greater patient choice and implementation of new booking systems (DH, 2002a, b). The introduction of new Diagnostic and Treatment Centres in England was also hailed as a means by which capacity could be increased within the NHS, providing opportunity for an additional 250 000 operations to occur by the end of 2005 (Beesley and Pirie, 2004; DH, 2002b). Government investment in day surgery provision proved popular with patients, NHS managers, clinicians and the DH alike and though reasons for doing so will differ, all parties extol the benefits of day surgery (DH, 2002a). All studies undertaken so far indicate a high level of patient satisfaction with the service; in fact the audit commission's report entitled 'Measuring Quality: The Patients' View of Day Surgery' (1991) demonstrated that 80% of patients were happy with the service.

From the patient's perspective there are numerous advantages to surgery on a day case basis, most particularly where day surgery does occur in a stand-alone or purpose-built unit. For example, the risk that a bed will not be available on the morning of surgery is removed, as is the risk that a more urgent case will take precedence. Additionally, day surgery provides the opportunity for recovery in one's own home, with less time in hospital resulting in less time to contract a hospital-acquired infection (HAI). There is minimal disruption to family life, and day surgery provides a much less daunting experience than an inpatient stay for those afraid of hospitals. For NHS managers, day surgery provides a cost-effective option since the need for expensive overnight accommodation is removed, acute beds are freed up and 'throughput' targets can be met. Clinicians appreciate day surgery because a fast turnover of patients' results in reduced waiting lists, shorter waiting times for operation, fewer cancellations and more sociable working hours.

However, popular as day surgery was seen to be, the efficiency of the service was questionable. A national study established that two-thirds of all day surgery cancellations resulted from patients cancelling themselves, often near to the time of surgery. This has huge ramifications for the effective use of theatre lists and theatre utilisation, particularly when late cancellations result in theatre slots remaining unoccupied (DH, 2002a). The extent of last-minute self-cancellations suggests a number of patients experience great uncertainty and apprehension regarding their forthcoming operation and the possibility that improved information giving and alleviation of uncertainty and apprehension could result in lower attrition rates. More detailed discussion with patients regarding the proposed surgery, taking account of preferred dates for surgery, special requirements associated with admission, the surgery itself and discharge support, could lessen preoperative anxiety and perhaps prevent many cancellations (NHS Modernisation Agency, 2002).

Hence, *effective* preoperative assessment is seen to be essential in minimising cancellations and in providing an efficient service responsive to the needs of the patient, as well as the organisation. Most NHS trusts now appreciate the importance of nurse-led pre-assessment in day surgery and have a strong commitment to staff development in order to improve the service delivered. The aim of this chapter is therefore to give an overview of the pre-assessment process, the role and responsibilities of the effective pre-assessment practitioner and the skills needed to assess patient suitability for day surgery.

The aims of preoperative assessment

One of the most important aims of pre-assessment is to establish that the patient fully understands the proposed procedure. Sometimes it could be said that the surgeon's and the patient's view of what is to be undertaken are 'at variance'. Therefore it is essential at pre-assessment that along with a thorough explanation of the procedure itself, the patient is given a clear indication of what to expect during his/her *perioperative* journey, from admission, through theatre, recovery and at discharge. It is important to remember that providing the patient with a comprehensive explanation and the opportunity to ask questions is fundamental to relieving anxiety and minimising fears, and following this discussion, it will be necessary for the patient to confirm verbally that he/she desires to proceed with the operation.

Reflection

At this point it might be useful to reflect on some of the issues and strategies surrounding communication and the ethical aspects of care discussed in Chapter 2.

Since not all oral information is retained in a stressful interview situation, it is helpful to provide additional written information in the form of patient information leaflets. Both patients and relatives find this form of communication useful to refer to whilst awaiting the proposed surgery. Often very specific instructions are given to patients with regard to such issues as preoperative fasting or bowel preparation. It may be helpful to jot these instructions down for patients. A contact telephone number should be given and the patient encouraged to communicate with the day surgery unit should they have additional queries or if it becomes necessary to cancel the operation.

There are risks associated with both surgery and anaesthesia. When the two are combined, the risks become proportionately greater. It is therefore essential to establish not only that the patient is fit to undergo surgery and well enough to receive an anaesthetic, but also that he/she will be able to tolerate the effects when both are combined (NHS Modernisation Agency, 2002). It is not cost effective for every day surgery unit to purchase instruments used on a very infrequent basis. Therefore on occasions highly specialised equipment or instrument sets must be ordered in. This is particularly the case for specialist orthopaedic instruments which may be hired from the manufacturer or loaned from another hospital. One of the aims of pre-assessment is to identify occasions when this is necessary. The skilled pre-assessment practitioner will be able to identify those patients for whom additional resources will be necessary and will communicate this to the theatre team.

Strict criteria must be met before the patient is deemed suitable for treatment within a day surgery unit, so careful history taking is important, as are the recording of baseline observations. Discussions regarding diet and lifestyle are in order when dealing with obese patients and those with diabetes and/or cardiovascular disease. Outcomes for patients who smoke and those who are obese can be improved with appropriate advice regarding weight loss and smoking cessation. With the current obesity epidemic and the recognised detrimental effects of obesity on the body, the opportunity for health promotion should never be missed (Cancer Research UK, 2006; Highfield, 2007).

If it is established during the pre-assessment process that the patient has difficulty in communicating, e.g. due to deafness, then this should be clearly indicated within the patient's notes. Individuals who do not have English as their first language may be accompanied by an interpreter. The need for an interpreter during the perioperative period should be documented along with any other individual needs or cultural requirements identified during the pre-assessment process. Finally, thought must be given to planning for discharge from hospital; therefore, the patient is questioned regarding travel arrangements and the support and home facilities available to them on discharge (NHS Modernisation Agency, 2005).

Thus it can be seen that the pre-assessment process is both detailed and comprehensive and is undertaken with the aim of ensuring a safe experience for the patient in conjunction with the smooth and efficient running of the theatre list. The NHS Modernisation Agency (2002) appropriately states:

> Preoperative assessment should lead to a fully prepared patient arriving fully prepared for surgery (p. 3).

The importance of effective preoperative assessment

Effective preoperative assessment was seen to be fundamental to improving hospital efficiency. As a result the NHS Modernisation Agency's Preoperative Assessment Project was designed to establish the way in which pre-assessment was conducted in many hospitals, with a view to subsequently developing and testing improvements. Nine NHS pilot sites were used in the study and the source of all day case cancellations was established (Figure 6.1). The study demonstrated that patients cancelling themselves accounted for approximately two-thirds of all cancellations occurring in day surgery, which has significant cost and efficiency implications, particularly

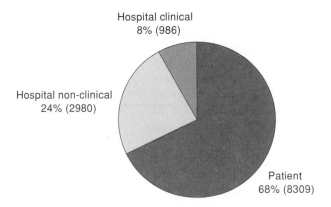

Figure 6.1   Source of all day-case cancellations. August 01–June 02. [NHS Modernisation Agency, 2002, p. 2, reproduced under the terms of the Click-Use Licence.]

where cancellations occur so close to the scheduled surgery that it proves impossible to fill vacant slots. In light of this, the study established reasons for day case cancellations on the day of, and the day before, surgery (Figure 6.2) (NHS Modernisation Agency, 2002).

The majority of late cancellations comprise patients who simply fail to attend on the day of surgery. Those who do contact the day surgery unit to inform staff of their decision not to attend for surgery give a variety of reasons, including inconvenient appointment times, feeling unfit for the proposed surgery or the operation being no longer required (NHS Modernisation Agency, 2002). Reasons for not attending for day surgery may well be genuine. However, there is the likelihood that many last-minute cancellations result from apprehension or uncertainty about the forthcoming procedure or aftercare, and this is sufficient to deter some from attending. The project highlighted that the implementation of effective preoperative assessment would, in particular, reduce the number of patients who simply did not attend (DNAs). Hence it is the *quality* of the preoperative assessment process which will make a difference in the full utilisation of theatre lists by reducing the number of last-minute cancellations. Preoperative assessment must therefore allow time for thorough discussion regarding the proposed surgery, which will do much to alleviate anxiety and apprehension. Patient choice regarding the convenience of the admission date must also be taken into account (NHS Modernisation Agency, 2002).

When and where pre-assessment takes place

New booking systems exist within primary care. Following a decision by the general practitioner (GP) that referral is necessary, the patient may access the 'Choose and Book' system which enables a choice between four hospitals, with an initial

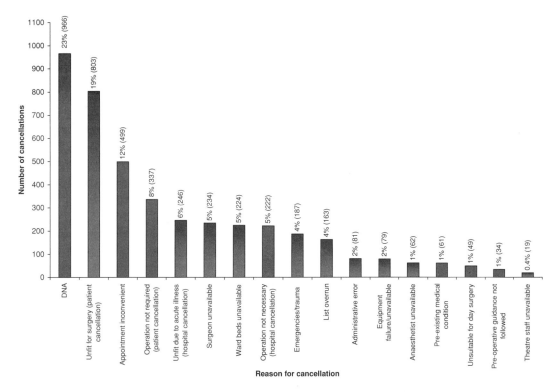

Figure 6.2 Reasons for day case cancellations on the day and the day before surgery. August 01–June 02. [NHS Modernisation Agency, 2002, p. 3, reproduced under the terms of the Click-Use Licence.]

outpatient appointment at a venue, time and date convenient to the individual. This can be undertaken immediately, within the GP surgery; alternatively the patient may choose to do this at a more convenient time using either phone or internet (NHS, 2007). According to 'National Good Practice Guidance on Preoperative Assessment for Day Surgery', pre-assessment is best undertaken during the initial consultation visit, directly after the decision to operate is made, thus ensuring a 'one-stop service' (NHS Modernisation Agency, 2002, p. 6).

This will be convenient to some because it obviates the need for a second hospital visit, thereby minimising travel and time costs. However, some individuals may consider themselves to be bombarded with information, entering the pre-assessment interview confused and bewildered and leaving the outpatient department in a similar manner (Edmondson, 1996). Additionally, in some instances and particularly where the appointment is related to the possibility of a diagnosis of cancer, the patient has insufficient time to come to terms with the need for surgery and, certainly, inadequate time to formulate questions.

Where consultants now sometimes undertake 'outreach' clinics within primary care, patient pre-assessment can be undertaken during the same visit. Other options for conducting preoperative assessment include the telephone via NHS

Direct or through the use of an internet questionnaire (NHS Modernisation Agency, 2005). The latter are particularly useful when more than 3 months have elapsed since pre-assessment took place, in which case the possibility of changes in the patient's condition dictates that 'reassessment' will be necessary prior to surgery.

Providing the normal processes are undertaken, exactly where pre-assessment takes place does not seem to be an important issue (DH, 2002a). However, those working in pre-assessment would recommend that the 20- to 30-min interview is undertaken within 3 months of the proposed surgery, at a designated day surgery unit. This allows the opportunity for patients to view the premises prior to surgery, which is both helpful and reassuring (Edmondson, 1996; Hodge, 1999). Preoperative assessment must always take place in a consultation room equipped with:

- Phlebotomy equipment
- An electrocardiograph (ECG) machine
- Sphygmomanometer (blood pressure machine)
- Weighing scales
- Some means of measuring the patient's height

The room must be away from patients recovering from surgery and completely private in order that patients feel able to ask and answer embarrassing or confidential questions. An engaged sign must be available to discourage interruptions during the assessment and examination processes.

Who should undertake the pre-assessment role and what skills are needed?

Historically the pre-assessment of patients was regarded as the province of the junior doctor; however, a 1992 audit commission report highlighted that where nurses adopted the pre-assessment role, improvements in the service were noted with fewer problems on the day of surgery and decreased DNA rates (Fysh, 1999). Pre-assessment by nurses may be more effective because they have more time for the interview, but also because medical staff may not take the patient's social situation into consideration. Additionally, nurses are seen to be more approachable, less intimidating, to have better communication skills and are more likely to be of the same social status as the patient (Edmondson, 1996; Fysh, 1999; Irvine et al., 1995).

The Royal College of Surgeons (1992) recognised the importance of the nurses' role in pre-assessment, highlighting that by ensuring patient fitness for surgery and anaesthesia, minimising patient cancellations and unplanned admissions nurses were making an invaluable contribution to efficiency within day surgery units (Janke et al., 2002; Markandy, 1997). For a variety of reasons then, nurses would appear to have adopted the role of preoperative assessment of patients undergoing day surgery, though other allied health professionals; e.g. operating department practitioners (ODPs) are equally suitable (NHS Modernisation Agency, 2002).

The importance of a multidisciplinary approach to patient selection cannot be overestimated since surgeons are often overly optimistic when deciding which patients are suitable for day surgery (McMillan, 2005). Certainly with the success of day surgery and increasing confidence on the part of the surgeon, referrals tend to be less cautious than previously (Edmondson, 1996). Those undertaking the pre-assessment role should, therefore, be experienced, assertive, competent practitioners specifically trained in pre-assessment. Currently the morbidity rate (measured, for example, in terms of poorly controlled pain, nausea or an unplanned overnight stay) associated with day surgery is 0.15%. Along with strict adherence to locally and nationally agreed guidelines for pre-assessment in day surgery, the pre-assessment practitioner should be adept at identifying those patients who may be at increased risk of complications, such as postoperative nausea and vomiting (PONV). Early identification can lead to effective management and this can significantly reduce the risk and complications associated with surgery (NHS Modernisation Agency, 2002, 2005).

Generally at pre-assessment there is no necessity for the patient to be examined by an anaesthetist; this can occur on the day of surgery. However, anaesthetic support, advice and guidance must be available to the pre-assessment practitioner, in order that potential problems can be identified and dealt with in advance of admission. Notes tend to be scrutinised by the pre-assessment practitioner the day before the patient's interview, and where necessary, anaesthetic opinion is sought in advance of the patient's appointment. The anaesthetist will be responsible for making a decision regarding the suitability of a patient once referred (Janke et al., 2002). Thoroughness and good decision-making skills are therefore a prerequisite of the pre-assessment practitioner, along with the ability to work closely with the medical team.

Health care practitioners can be prepared for the pre-assessment role by participation in appropriate educational and experiential training programmes, and both in-house and university-based accredited courses specific to day surgery are currently available (Fysh, 1999). In 2002, the Operating Theatre and Preoperative Assessment Programme commissioned a CD rom and training manual on preoperative assessment from Southampton University. 'Setting a Standard through Learning' allows medical students, doctors in training, nurses and allied health professionals to undertake comprehensive in-house training in pre-assessment. Interested readers can obtain the package by Janke et al. (2002) through an inter-library loan from Southampton University.

When health care professionals are initially acquiring pre-assessment skills, careful observation of experienced practitioners is necessary for several weeks. A period of supported practice is then required, with the trainee undertaking the pre-assessment interview and the expert practitioner contributing only when supplementary information is necessary or advice is requested. Following on from this, the health care professional can undertake unsupervised pre-assessment interviews, but with the reassurance of indirect support provided by more experienced practitioners simultaneously conducting pre-assessment interviews within the department.

The prospect of surgery is for most individuals, a stressor which will provoke anxiety. The ready availability of medical information via the internet has resulted in many patients arriving at pre-assessment already well informed about their condition; it is indeed the era of the 'expert patient'. Even when the proposed procedure is relatively minor, most patients are only too aware of the risks associated with administration of a general anaesthetic and some may express fears of dying during surgery (Rogan Foy and Timmins, 2004). Pain, a threat to body image through scars and deformities, fear of an unknown environment and potential mistakes in documentation also give cause for anxiety (Lock, 1999). Fyffe (1999) examined some of the factors commonly serving to act as stressors to patients; along with death, many patients verbalised fears that they will be awake and experience pain during the procedure, that the wrong part of the body may be operated on or that they may not recover from anaesthesia.

So far within this text it has been emphasised that the giving of verbal and written information during pre-assessment can do much to reduce anxiety and stress and reduce DNA rates. Better preparation of patients may result in faster recovery from anaesthesia and a reduction in the experience of postoperative pain (Fyffe, 1999; NHS Modernisation Agency, 2002). Grieve (2002) however considers that

> ... anxiety-reduction is being overshadowed by uncertainty-reduction approaches which place a disproportionate emphasis on the provision of information (p. 670).

In his examination of preoperative anxiety-reduction and coping strategies of patients undergoing day surgery, Grieve (2002, p. 671) makes reference to the work of Krohne et al. (1996), who identify two groups of patients. *Vigilant copers* are those patients who will want to know absolutely everything about their operation: what will be involved, how they will feel afterwards and who actively employ coping mechanisms. *Avoidance copers* on the other hand will tend to employ passive coping mechanisms desiring the minimum amount of information necessary to proceed with their operation and preferring generally not to think about it. In reality, these coping strategies will not be exclusive but probably represent opposing ends of a continuum with an individual's coping mechanisms determining his/her place on the continuum.

The essence of Grieve's work is to emphasise that for some individuals, the giving of verbal and written information may serve to increase anxiety rather than to alleviate it, and as a result, he places greater importance on the true therapeutic potential of the nurse–patient relationship to reduce anxiety, which, he states, is underappreciated by nurses. The relevance of referring to Grieve's work here is to highlight that *what becomes routine for the pre-assessment practitioner is not routine for the patient*. Information giving should therefore be individualised, and the pre-assessment practitioner needs to become adept at assessing how much information the patient really wants. This idea reflects the stance taken in the chapter on communication where empowering the patient is about the patient defining what is in his/her best interests.

Since surgery may be of an embarrassing and/or sensitive nature, pre-assessment practitioners need to develop skills enabling them to put the patient at ease. An empathic attitude is another prerequisite of the role, as is conveying an air of professionalism and confidence. Significant knowledge of anatomy, physiology and the surgical procedures undertaken within the department are crucial. Due to the short duration of the interview, finely honed communication skills are fundamental to developing the therapeutic relationship necessary between pre-assessor and patient (Rogan Foy and Timmins, 2004; Wicker and O'Neil, 2006). Communication skills can be learnt, and the pre-assessment practitioner should be well versed in the use of verbal and non-verbal communication skills, the use of open and closed questions to elicit appropriate information and, equally importantly, demonstrate active listening skills (Rogan Foy and Timmins, 2004).

Cumulative knowledge

Visit Chapter 2 and refresh your knowledge regarding communication skills. Identify those pertinent to preoperative assessment.

Meeting the criteria necessary for surgery within a day surgery unit

In 1990, the Audit Commission working in consultation with BADS specified 20 procedures suitable for undertaking within a day surgery unit, placing them in a metaphorical supermarket 'trolley'. Continuing the analogy, in 2001, a further 'basket' of procedures was added to the trolley, with recommendations that as many as possible of these specified procedures should be undertaken on a day case basis (DH, 2002a).

However, patients are not selected for day surgery purely because the procedure they are to undergo is included in the 'trolley'; other operations may still be suitable for undertaking within a day surgery unit, and all patients must meet certain criteria. Physical health is assessed along with social circumstances, and lastly, the patient must be in agreement with receiving surgery on a day case basis. Recommendations are that any patient undergoing an appropriate procedure should be considered for day surgery; and only if full preoperative assessment demonstrates a contraindication, should they be excluded. Indeed the new maxim should be:

Is there any justification for admitting this patient as an in-patient? (DH, 2002a, p. 6).

Commencement of the day surgery selection process usually begins with referral of the patient following initial consultation in an outpatient or outreach clinic. Providing the consultant deems the procedure suitable for day surgery; the patient will either be placed on a waiting list for preoperative assessment to be undertaken or referred directly to the day surgery unit for pre-assessment. It will be the responsibility of the pre-assessment practitioner to be clear and objective in determining both the procedure and patient's suitability for day surgery. If the procedure meets the following criteria, then it will usually be considered suitable:

- In general, a procedure of $1^1/_2$-hour duration or less. (Invasiveness must be assessed if the procedure is anticipated to take longer than 1 hour.)
- Pain on discharge must be controllable with oral analgesia.
- Minimal or no risk of continued blood loss following surgery, nor anticipation of homeostatic imbalance affecting cardiac or respiratory systems.
- No interruption of blood flow to major organs expected.
- Intravenous fluids will be unnecessary postoperatively.
- No open cases (as opposed to a laparoscopic approach) involving the thoracic or abdominal cavities (though mini laparotomies, for example, for sterilisation would be possible) (NHS Modernisation Agency, 2002; McMillan, 2005).

If the patient chooses not to have their surgery on a day case basis, personal preference is respected and referral to an inpatient list is made. On the whole, patients are happy to participate in day surgery and subsequently receive a letter giving notification of a 'pre-assessment' interview date. Often a health questionnaire, which serves as an early warning system for patients with complex medical needs, is administered to patients when first placed on the waiting list. Alternatively, this may be completed by the patient when first arriving for pre-assessment (Jackson, 2004).

At pre-assessment itself, an additional questionnaire is completed in consultation with the pre-assessment practitioner who then documents the patient's medical condition and social circumstances. The questionnaire normally forms part of an integrated care pathway (ICP), which is a tool designed at local level by the multidisciplinary team, based on evidence and guidelines, for use throughout the patient's journey.

The ICP usually takes the form of a booklet which will constitute the clinical records of the patient, documenting the patient's medical history, clinical and personal details and the care received from admission through to discharge. There are many benefits to the implementation of ICPs in a day surgery setting, including facilitation of risk management, accurate record keeping and improved communication between the multidisciplinary team. As well as minimising repetition, referral to the ICP can ensure that the patient is not bothered with repetitive questions. The booklet is particularly useful for new, agency and locum staff, serving, as it does, as a specific framework or guide to follow (British Association of Day Surgery (BADS), 2004a; NHS Modernisation Agency, 2005).

Opportunity for the student

Check out the link to the BADS documentation website at
http://www.daysurgeryuk.org/content/Professionals/Documentation.asp

Here you will find a selection of care plans and ICPs which will give you considerable insight into the pre-assessment interview. Select an ICP and find the pre-assessment section detailing all the questions asked by the pre-assessment practitioner. Read through this, imagining yourself in the role of the pre-assessment practitioner.

Discussion regarding the patient's social circumstances is important in ascertaining whether adequate support will be available postoperatively. Lack of any of the following mean day surgery is contraindicated:

- An escort and the means of travelling home by taxi or private car
- A relative or friend (over 18 years of age) in good physical health, able to stay with the patient for 24 hours following sedation or a general anaesthetic
- Easy access to the home/overnight accommodation
- An indoor toilet
- Access to a telephone
- GP/nursing backup

Enquiries should also be made regarding dependent relatives and young children, since it is not appropriate to discharge patients to an environment where they may have to look after others. A journey of more than 1 hour following the surgery may also be a contraindication, although this depends on the type of surgery undertaken and the availability of local medical assistance. An explanation must be given that a prolonged journey time may increase the risk of nausea, vomiting and pain. Providing the patient understands and is happy to take the risk and careful documentation of discussions occurs, then day surgery may proceed. If a patient is unable to comply with the criteria outlined above, he/she may be referred for inpatient treatment, or where hospital hotel services are available to a trust, these may be utilised (Fysh, 1999; NHS Modernisation Agency, 2005).

The patient's general health and fitness for surgery and anaesthesia will be ascertained. In the main, age does not preclude anyone from day surgery, although local policy will determine the lowest age limit. (Often infants below 6 months will receive treatment within a specialist unit.) Whilst it is recognised that there are a higher proportion of cardiovascular events in those over 65, the patient's biological condition rather than chronological age should be the determining factor (Chung et al., 1999).

The American Society of Anesthesiologists (ASA) devised an assessment tool whereby a patient's physical status and suitability for anaesthesia (based on past medical and anaesthetic history) could be classified (Box 6.1).

Box 6.1 American Society of Anesthesiologists (ASA) physical status grade

---

(1) Healthy patient. Localised surgical pathology with no systemic disturbance
(2) Mild/moderate systemic disturbance (the surgical pathology or other disease process). No activity limitation
(3) Severe systemic disturbance from any cause. Some activity limitation
(4) Life-threatening systemic disorder. Severe activity limitation
(5) Moribund patient with little chance of survival

NHS Modernisation Agency (2002, p. 12), reproduced under the terms of the Click-Use Licence.

Use of the ASA descriptors (the 'ASA status') allows instant and easy recognition of patient's physical health. This is extremely useful in surgery for documentation purposes and particularly so in day surgery. Formerly, ASA 1 and ASA 2 patients would be accepted for day surgery; however, improvements in anaesthetic and surgical techniques have been considerable in recent years and as a result, it is now commonplace for ASA 3 patients to be accepted for day surgery, unless the pre-assessment process highlights contraindications (NHS Modernisation Agency, 2002). Therefore, pre-assessment of ASA 3 patients must be a rigorous process whereby it is established that systemic disease is well controlled. Inappropriate patient selection can result in unplanned admissions to inpatient wards, increased complications and increased anaesthetic and nursing time (Fysh, 1999). The smooth running of the operating list and day surgery unit can, therefore, be compromised.

The pre-assessment practitioner will record baseline readings of pulse and blood pressure, and height and weight are documented. Body mass index (BMI) is established and the patient's medical status assessed, with relevant comorbidities (e.g. well-controlled diabetes) documented. If a contraindication to day surgery is established (e.g. unstable diabetes), referral to an inpatient list should occur (BADS, 2004b). Current medications are recorded along with allergies and advice is given regarding discontinuation of herbal medications 2 weeks prior to surgery since these can have side effects when combined with surgery and/or anaesthesia. Most organisations have developed local thrombosis risk score charts, and the patient's risk of developing a deep vein thrombosis is assessed by the pre-assessment practitioner.

The patient is questioned regarding personal experience or family history of problematic anaesthesia, and assessment of the airway and mobility of the neck is conducted (Janke et al., 2002). The patient will be asked to open the mouth as wide as possible and fully extend the tongue. Ideally the pharyngeal pillars, soft palate and uvula will be visible. This will be rated as Class 1 on the Mallampati pharyngeal assessment scale (Figure 6.3), with a view of only the soft palate and uvula rated as Class 2 (NHS Modernisation Agency, 2002). Both are considered suitable for day surgery. If a patient has very limited mouth opening, is unable to open the mouth or has a history of difficult *intubation*, then he/she will be precluded from day surgery. Relative contraindications to day surgery are those patients with a receding jaw, short fat neck, restricted mouth opening or those classed as 3 (soft palate only visible) or 4 (soft palate not visible) on the Mallampati scale. Referral to an anaesthetist will then be necessary (NHS Modernisation Agency, 2002).

Patients needing additional investigation/referral

Patients with arthritis of the cervical spine or mandible problems which would make neck extension and intubation difficult require investigation by the anaesthetist, as will those with a history of anaesthetic problems. Patients with unstable conditions such as uncontrolled epilepsy, diabetes or hypertension are not suitable for day surgery and will be referred to an inpatient list. Obese patients, those with a history of stroke, transient ischaemic attacks, asthma, respiratory or cardiac disease, will necessitate very careful investigation and, where necessary, further investigations or referral will be organised.

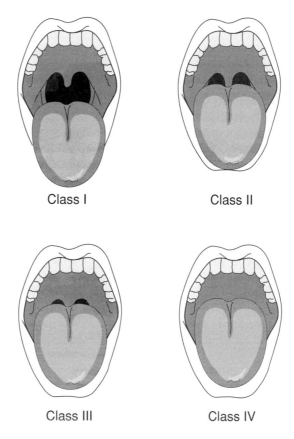

Figure 6.3 Mallampati classification for difficult intubation. [Reproduced from Berry and Kohn's *Operating Room Technique*, 10th ed., Phillips, 2004, p. 405, with permission from Elsevier.]

Body mass index

Patients whose BMI is below 35 will be accepted for day surgery. Patients with a BMI between 35 and 40 kg/m^2 will be accepted for the majority of procedures in most day surgery units. The BMI (measured as weight in kilograms divided by height in metres squared) is not always representative of a patient's suitability for day surgery as athletes and bodybuilders have a high BMI but none of the relevant comorbidity associated with obesity. Laparoscopic procedures and hernia repairs become progressively more difficult with increased abdominal fat; therefore, waist measurement gives a more accurate indication of the suitability of the individual for surgery, with the thinner abdomen of a 'pear-shaped' individual being preferable to that of a larger 'apple shape' (BADS, 2004c; McMillan, 2005). Since health promotion is included in the role of the pre-assessment practitioner, it would be in order to discuss weight loss strategies with the patient and suggest referral to a weight-loss clinic or dietitian.

Hypertension

Hypertension can be a predictor of postoperative myocardial infarction and is associated with increased morbidity and complications when the condition is not well controlled prior to surgery (McMillan, 2005). A raised blood pressure at interview may be the result of anxiety and remonitoring 10–20 min later is advisable. A continued raised blood pressure necessitates referral back to the patient's GP. A standardised proforma indicating the need for surgery complicated by the raised blood pressure is completed and signed by the pre-assessment practitioner. Hand delivery of the letter to the GP surgery and arrangement of a prompt appointment is recommended to the patient.

Depending on the closeness of the date of surgery, it may be necessary to reschedule to allow time for stabilisation of the blood pressure. Patients are asked to make contact with the day surgery unit when their GP deems the blood pressure suitably reduced. Generally, antihypertensive medication must be taken on the day of surgery (McMillan, 2005). However, angiotensin-converting enzyme (ACE) inhibitors (which all end with 'pril', e.g. ramipril), angiotensin II receptor antagonists (which usually end with 'sartan', e.g. candesartan) and doxazocin must be withheld on the day of surgery. In combination with anaesthesia these drugs cause profound hypotension.

Diabetes

Patients with diabetes are not precluded from day surgery, provided their disease is well controlled. Scheduling first on the operating list facilitates early return to eating, drinking and medication, and for the same reason, it is important that postoperative nausea and vomiting is minimised. For both Type 1 and Type 2 disease, breakfast and oral hypoglycaemic medication or insulin will be withheld when surgery takes place during a morning list. Providing the blood glucose is between 6 and 10 mmols, surgery proceeds. When scheduled for afternoon surgery, the anaesthetist will advise regarding fasting time and medication but, generally, breakfast and medication are taken (NHS Modernisation Agency, 2002; McMillan, 2005).

Opportunity for the student

BADS has produced detailed and useful guidance entitled 'Day Surgery and the Diabetic Patient' (2004b). This can be found at
http://www.daysurgeryuk.org/content/files/Handbooks/DaySurgeryDiabetic.pdf
    Access this information and answer the following critical review questions:

(1) Certain factors will exclude patients with diabetes from having surgery within a day surgery unit, what are they?
(2) When accepting the diabetic patient for day surgery, certain information regarding the patient's disease must be established. Establish exactly what the pre-assessment practitioner must investigate.

Asthma

While patients who are fit and have well-controlled asthma are accepted for day surgery; those requiring oral steroids on a frequent basis or those who have been recently hospitalised for treatment of their asthma may be contraindicated. Peak expiratory flow and spirometry tests will be useful in decision making and referral to the anaesthetist may be necessary.

Respiratory conditions

Patients with respiratory problems are graded on the amount of breathlessness they experience (Box 6.2). Dyspnoea of grades 0–2 are acceptable for day surgery; grades 3 and 4 are precluded as are patients with sleep apnoea (NHS Modernisation Agency, 2002).

Box 6.2 Dyspnoea grading

---

0. No dyspnoea whilst walking on level at normal pace.
1. Mild, non-specific (speed not distance) restriction. 'Walk as far as I like provided I take my time'.
2. Moderate, specific, outdoor limitation. 'Stop for a while after ... (a recognisable distance limitation')'.
3. Marked dyspnoea on mild, indoor exertion. 'Stop for a while between kitchen and bathroom'.
4. Incapacitation. Dyspnoea at rest.

NHS Modernisation Agency (2002, p. 13), reproduced under the terms of the Click-Use Licence.

Cardiac conditions

Patients with potentially treatable conditions may be suitable for day surgery once they have been referred and commenced treatment, at which time fitness will be reassessed. These conditions will include those with untreated angina classification 2 (Box 6.3), those with either uncontrolled or poorly controlled cardiac failure which results in grade 3 or 4 dyspnoea (Box 6.2) or those who are unable to sleep flat and wake at night gasping for breath (orthopnoea). Where patients are on warfarin or aspirin, it is possible to undertake some minor procedures but the surgeon must be contacted for advice. Referral to an anaesthetist is necessary where the patient has experienced either a transient ischaemic attack or a cerebrovascular incident during the past year (NHS Modernisation Agency, 2002).

Box 6.3 New York Heart Association classification of angina

0. No angina.
1. No limitation of ordinary physical activity. Angina caused by strenuous or rapid prolonged exertion.
2. Slight limitation of normal activity, e.g. angina with rapid walking, climbing stairs, emotional stress.
3. Marked limitation of normal activity, e.g. angina on one flight of stairs. Comfortable at rest.
4. Incapacitation. Angina on mildest effort or at rest.

NHS Modernisation Agency (2002, p. 14), reproduced under the terms of the Click-Use Licence.

Ordering further investigations

The undertaking of routine, blanket investigations prior to day surgery is seen to be unnecessary, inefficient and costly. Patients who are under 50 and in good health do not require routine investigations (NHS Modernisation Agency, 2002).

Opportunity for the student

The National Institute for Health and Clinical Excellence (NICE) (2003) developed comprehensive clinical guidelines regarding the preoperative tests necessary for patients undergoing elective surgery of a minor, intermediate, major and major+ nature. This is available at http://www.nice.org.uk/pdf/CG3NICEguideline.pdf

It would be useful to access this information with a view to determining the investigations necessary for children and adults undergoing all forms of surgery.

Most departments have established protocols indicating the type of investigations to be ordered in specific situations, though recent test results will obviate the need for repetition (within 3 months unless changes in the patient's clinical condition have occurred). Existing and newly ordered investigation results need to be carefully examined by the pre-assessment team in order that decisions regarding patient management can be made (Janke et al., 2002). Only a brief overview indicating the conditions for which specific investigations are needed is possible here:

- Urinalysis
  - Undertaken on all patients
- ECG
  - Over 50 years
  - Chest pain/palpitations/collapse/dizziness
  - Hypertension
  - Respiratory disease, heavy smoker
  - Heart murmur/carotid bruits/cardiac disease

- Respiratory disease
- History of myocardial infarction
- Morbid obesity (BMI over 38)
- Diabetes
- Electrolytes, creatinine
  - Hypertension
  - Diabetes
  - Renal disease
  - Diuretic treatment
  - Cardiac disease
  - Patients over 60
  - Patients on steroids
- Full blood count
  - Termination of pregnancy
  - Evacuation of retained products of conception (ERPC)
  - Anaemia, ulcerative colitis, Crohn's disease, rheumatoid arthritis
  - Menorrhagia
  - Long-term non-steroidal anti-inflammatory drug use
  - Malignancy
  - Liver disease
  - Abnormal bleeding
  - Chronic disease states
  - Patients over 60
  - Patients on anticoagulants
- Group and save
  - Termination of pregnancy
  - Evacuation of retained products of conception (ERPC)
  - Laparoscopic cholecystectomy
- Sickle-cell test
  - Afro-Caribbean extraction (may carry status card)
- Thyroid function test
  - Breathlessness of recent onset
  - Atrial fibrillation
  - Hypo/hyperthyroidism
- Liver function test
  - Adult jaundice
  - High alcohol intake (>40 units per week)
  - Cholecystectomy/hepatobiliary surgery
  - Drug abuse
- Respiratory function tests
  - Recent increased breathlessness
- Clotting studies
  - Laparoscopic cholecystectomy
  - History of bleeding
  - Liver disease
  - Renal disease

(NHS Modernisation Agency, 2002; McMillan, 2005)

Giving information to patients

Towards the end of the interview it will be necessary for the pre-assessment practitioner to check that the patient has been given information regarding the following:

- An explanation of the procedure (with written information if available)
- Fasting time and any other preoperative preparation necessary, e.g. bowel preparation or suppositories
- An idea of the level of discomfort which will be experienced and the pain relief available
- Possible side effects and action to be taken
- An approximation of the time away from work
- Advice regarding when to resume driving and other usual activities
- A contact number for the patient to ring in the event that:
  - He/she cannot attend for surgery
  - A significant change to the patient's medical condition has occurred
  - There have been changes to the patient's drug regime
  - Advice is needed
- An indication of what the patient will need to bring on the actual day of admission, e.g. medication and slippers
- Parking and dropping off areas
- Whether it is possible to be accompanied by relatives
  (NHS Modernisation Agency, 2002)

Reasons for reassessment

Those patients who undergo surgery within 3 months of pre-assessment are unlikely to need reassessment unless a change in condition occurs. If surgery does not occur within 3 months then reassessment will be necessary as changes in the patient's condition and medication may have occurred, and blood tests would need repeating. Additionally, information given to the patient may have been forgotten. Reassessment may also be necessary if the patient has experienced a hospital admission, undergoes new treatment or perhaps has a minor illness affecting them on the scheduled date of surgery.

Auditing the service

The purpose of audit is to ensure continual improvement of the service delivered to patients. Generally, patients are telephoned the day after discharge to check whether any problems are being encountered. This service provides considerable reassurance to individuals, allowing questions to be asked. Patient satisfaction with the service and unacceptable morbidity levels experienced at home can be ascertained at this time. Day surgery throughput should be collated including attendees and non-attendees for pre-assessment; non-attendees for surgery and unplanned overnight stays. Reasons for the cancellation of operations by both the hospital and the patient should be investigated further (NHS Modernisation Agency, 2002).

Scenario

Mrs Green has been referred from the breast clinic for excision of a wire localisation of breast lesion. She has attended pre-assessment prior to receiving her appointment for day surgery, along with her husband. Mrs Green seems distracted and extremely anxious about the speed with which events are unfolding, particularly since she is unable to feel the lump. Breast lumps can be difficult to detect due to position in the breast, size and consistency. However, in some instances they become X-ray detectable before becoming palpable by the patient or surgeon. X-ray localisation of the lesion and insertion of a guide-wire prior to surgery will help in identification of the mass at the time of the operation.

(1) Do you think Mrs Green is going to have a number of questions as yet unanswered? If so, which skills will be employed by the pre-assessment practitioner in order to deal with them?

(2) Holistic care incorporates support of the immediate family. The fact that Mr Green is in attendance indicates family involvement, but how much does Mr Green know and how much does Mrs Green want him to know about her treatment? How can this be established?

(3) Empathy is essential when dealing with patients newly diagnosed with cancer. Can you imagine yourself in Mrs Green's situation and how will this help in your interactions with her?

Summary

In recent years, there has been enormous political pressure to reduce waiting lists, waiting times and cancelled operations and to improve the patient's experience of surgery. Day surgery is seen as being a major part of the solution. This overview of the pre-assessment process has highlighted the importance of *effective* pre-assessment in reducing patient cancellations. The pre-assessment practitioner has a fundamental role in reducing patient anxiety; therefore, excellent communication skills are paramount. Determining a patient's suitability for surgery and anaesthesia carries with it enormous responsibility due to the autonomy inherent within the role; therefore, the importance of pre-assessment within day surgery cannot be overestimated.

Acknowledgement

While the author is responsible for the text, she thanks Liz Gregson, pre-assessment sister at Queen Elizabeth the Queen Mother Hospital at Margate in Kent for checking the accuracy of the work.

Glossary of terms

Intubation
This process occurs as the patient is being anaesthetised and involves insertion of a plastic tube into the patient's oral or nasal passageway to ensure adequate and safe ventilation during surgery. Securing of the airway allows administration of inhalational agents during the procedure (see Chapter 9).

Perioperative
This encompasses the various stages within the patient's journey through surgery, commencing with admission, through the induction of anaesthesia, surgery, recovery, the immediate postoperative period right through to discharge.

Websites

British Association of Day Surgery (No date given) Documentation Website. Available from:
http://www.daysurgeryuk.org/content/Professionals/Documentation.asp (accessed 14 June 2007).

References

Beesley, J. and Pirie, S. (eds) (2004) *NATN Standards and Recommendations for Safe Perioperative Practice*. UK: National Association of Theatre Nurses.

British Association of Day Surgery (BADS) (2004a) *Integrated Care Pathways for Day Surgery Patients*. Available from: http://www.daysurgeryuk.org/content/Professionals/Documentation.asp (accessed 4 April 2007).

British Association of Day Surgery (BADS) (2004b) *Day Surgery and the Diabetic Patient*. Available from: http://www.daysurgeryuk.org/content/files/Handbooks/DaySurgeryDiabetic.pdf (accessed 26 June 2007).

British Association of Day Surgery (BADS) (2004c) *Day Case Laparoscopic Cholecystectomy*. Available from: http://www.daysurgeryuk.org/content/Professionals/BADS-Handbooks.asp (accessed 4 May 2007).

British Association of Day Surgery (BADS) (n.d.) Documentation website. Available from: http://www.daysurgeryuk.org/content/Professionals/Documentation.asp (accessed 14 June 2007).

Cancer Research UK (2006) Britain warned that obesity will cause thousands more cases of cancer. Available from: http://science.cancerresearchuk.org/news/archivednews/obesity_epidemic?version=1 (accessed 12 September 2007).

Chung, F., Mezei, R. and Tong, D. (1999) Adverse events in ambulatory surgery. A comparison between elderly and younger patients. *Canadian Journal of Anaesthesiology 46*, pp. 309–321.

Edmondson, M. (1996) Day surgery, in Penn, S., Davenport, H.T., Carrington, S. and Edmondson, M. (eds) *Principles of Day Surgery Nursing*. Great Britain: Blackwell Science Ltd, pp. 37–61.

Fyffe, A. (1999) Anxiety and the preoperative patient. *British Journal of Theatre Nursing* 9(10), pp. 452–454.

Fysh, R. (1999) Patient selection, in Hodge, D. (ed) *Day Surgery. A Nursing Approach*. London: Churchhill Livingstone, pp. 5–25.

Department of Health (DH) (2000) *The NHS Plan: Creating a 21st Century*. NHS. London: HMSO.

Department of Health (DH) (2002a) *Day Surgery: Operational Guide*. UK: Department of Health Publications. Available from: http://www.dh.gov.uk/en/Policyandguidance/ Organisationpolicy/Secondarycare/Daysurgery/index.htm (accessed 24 March 2007).

Department of Health (DH) (2002b) *Thousands of NHS Patients to Benefit From Day Surgery Expansion – Hutton*. Available from: http://www.dh.gov.uk/en/ Publicationsandstatistics/Pressreleases/DH_4014344 (accessed 24 March 2007).

Grieve, R. (2002) Day surgery preoperative anxiety reduction and coping strategies. *British Journal of Nursing 11*(10), pp. 670–678.

Highfield, R. (6 June 2007) Microwave 'sparked obesity epidemic'. *Telegraph* [online]. Available from: http://www.telegraph.co.uk/news/main.jhtml?xml=/news/2007/06/ 06/nfood306.xml (accessed 12 September 2007).

Hodge, D. (1999) *Day Surgery – A Nursing Approach*. Edinburgh: Churchill Livingstone.

Irvine, C., White, J. and Ingoldby, C. (1995) Nurse screening before intermediate day case surgery. *Journal of One Day Surgery 4*(3), pp. 5–7.

Jackson, J. (2004) Safe admission. *Nursing Standard 19*(8), p. 14.

Janke, E., Chalk, V. and Kinley, H. (2002) *Preoperative Assessment: Setting A Standard Through Learning*. UK: University of Southampton.

Krohne, H., Slangen, K. and Kleeman, P. (1996) Coping variables as predictors of perioperative emotional states and adjustment. *Psychological Health 11*(3), pp. 315–330.

Lock, E. (1999) Preparation for procedures, in Hodge, D. (ed.) *Day Surgery – A Nursing Approach*. Edinburgh: Churchill Livingstone, pp. 27–39.

Markandy, L. (ed.) (1997) *Day Surgery for Nurses*. London: Whurr Publishers Ltd.

McMillan, R. (2005) Day surgery, in Woodhead, K. and Whicker, P. (eds) *A Textbook of Perioperative Care*. Philadelphia: Elsevier Churchill Livingstone, pp. 199–220.

NHS Modernisation Agency (2002) *National Good Practice Guidance on Preoperative Assessment for Day Surgery*. Available from: http://www.wise.nhs.uk/cmsWISE/ Cross+Cutting+Themes/access/elective/documents/documents.htm (accessed 9 April 2007).

NHS Modernisation Agency (2005) *Day Surgery – A Good Practice Guide*. Available from: http://www.wise.nhs.uk/cmsWISE/Cross+Cutting+Themes/access/elective/documents/ documents.htm (accessed 20 June 2007).

National Health Service (2007) "What is Choose and Book?" *Choose and Book Website*. Available from: http://www.chooseandbook.nhs.uk/staff/reference/choose-and-book-bulletins (accessed 11 April 2007).

National Institute for Health and Clinical Excellence (2003) *Preoperative Tests. The Use of Routine Preoperative Tests for Elective Surgery*. Available from: http://www.nice.org.uk/pdf/CG3NICEguideline.pdf (accessed 11 April 2007).

Rogan Foy, C. and Timmins, F. (2004) Improving communication in day surgery settings. *Nursing Standard 19*(7), pp. 37–42.

Royal College of Surgeons (1992) *Report of the Working Party on Guidelines for Day Case Surgery*. London: Royal College of Surgeons.

Wicker, P. and O'Neil, J. (2006) *Caring for the Perioperative Patient*. Oxford: Blackwell Publishing Ltd.

Further reading

McMillan, R. (2005) Day surgery, in Woodhead, K. and Wicker, P. *A Textbook of Perioperative Care*. Philadelphia: Elsevier Churchill Livingstone, pp. 199–220.

NHS Modernisation Agency (2002) *National Good Practice Guidance on Preoperative Assessment for Day Surgery*. Available from: http://www.wise.nhs.uk/cmsWISE/Cross+Cutting+Themes/access/elective/documents/documents.htm (accessed 9 April 2007).

Chapter 7

Radiology nursing

Lioba Howatson-Jones

Learning objectives
After reading this chapter the reader will be able to:

(1) Identify the role of the nurse in preparing and supporting the patient
(2) Demonstrate knowledge of health and safety concerns
(3) Describe a variety of imaging procedures
(4) Identify appropriate preparation and aftercare
(5) Describe potential complications and management strategies
(6) Consider future developments

Introduction

Definition

Radiology comprises a number of different imaging modalities that examine the structure and function of the body and apply treatments.

The medical impetus for minimally invasive interventions and the ability to undertake these under local anaesthetic or conscious sedation have driven progress of the radiological approach to many procedures (Watkinson et al., 2002). Innovations in imaging technology and equipment have led to increasingly complex treatments becoming available, reducing a patient's hospital stay. Radiology nurses provide care for patients undergoing imaging procedures. Department infrastructure makes this a rather public arena in which to carry out assessment and intimate examinations requiring advanced communication and advocacy skills. A variety of diverse staff are essential to carry out the procedures providing opportunities for inter-professional working and role progression. The critical practitioner maintains awareness of the multiple professional stances whilst engaging with their own practice development.

The chapter is divided into two sections. In part one issues related to radiology as a specialty are considered. The science of imaging modalities is explained and the use of various types of contrast for enhancing imaging is discussed in physiological terms. Health and safety are considered in terms of radiation risk, infection control and manual handling. Consent is explored in the context of relating to unknown long-term outcomes of evolving procedures and treatments. The role of the nurse in creating an atmosphere of trust, providing assistance and future role developments, is examined. In part two some general diagnostic and interventional procedures are considered in terms of care requirement and nursing input. It is not the intention of this text to provide a profile of every procedure but to consider the more common ones.

Part 1: Issues relating to radiology as a specialty

The science of imaging modalities

X-rays were discovered by Wilhelm Conrad Röntgen in 1895. X-rays are produced by electromagnetic particle waves accelerating towards a tungsten target. As they strike, electrons are disrupted and change their orbit around the atom nucleus releasing energy creating a photon, or X-ray beam, of radiation as illustrated in Figure 7.1. This happens in the X-ray tube of the machine.

Radiation is directed to penetrate matter, with some being absorbed by the body as the beam passes through, depending on the density of the tissue involved. For example, bone appears solid and white because the atoms are larger, soft tissue is moderately transparent because there is less absorption and air is completely transparent appearing black. The degree of absorption is called attenuation and outlines the structure as the beam is converted into light on an intensifier screen. This either exposes a photosensitive film to produce a hard copy or is read digitally producing a computer image. Continuous exposure produces an image in real time that can be

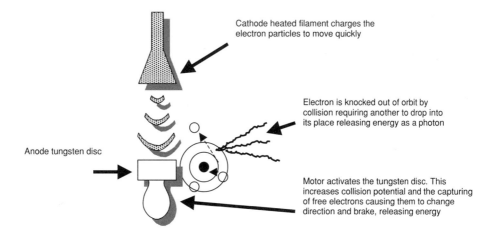

Cathode heated filament charges the electron particles to move quickly

Electron is knocked out of orbit by collision requiring another to drop into its place releasing energy as a photon

Anode tungsten disc

Motor activates the tungsten disc. This increases collision potential and the capturing of free electrons causing them to change direction and brake, releasing energy

Figure 7.1   How an X-ray is produced.

manipulated and magnified through computer technology for more detailed imaging of structures. This is called fluoroscopy and is displayed as a television image (Jones and Taylor, 2006). Radiation is dangerous in pregnancy, particularly in the first trimester when organs are forming, because of the attenuation factor that can alter cell DNA and result in mutations in the fetus.

Ultrasound uses high-frequency sound waves to penetrate body structures and the degree of echo received back is translated into a computer image. It is particularly useful for outlining internal organs and fluid collections. Hard tissues like bone reflect the most echoes and appear white. Soft tissues appear grey and speckled. Fluids do not reflect echoes and appear black. Abdominal scans require a full bladder to assist with differentiating structures. Probes may be used to assist with viewing internal structures such as the uterus and ovaries (transvaginal probe) and prostate (rectal probe). Because no radiation is involved this modality is safe to use during pregnancy.

Mammography utilises low-dose radiation X-rays to create an image of the internal structure of the breasts. Fat appears grey and glandular tissue white. It is particularly useful for highlighting developing problems that are asymptomatic at an early stage. Two views are taken to enable maximum orientation. Advancements have been made into digital mammography where X-rays are converted into electrical signals that are electronically detected, enabling computer and hard copy display within seconds rather than the minutes required for conventional film development. Computer-aided detection (CAD) utilises software that manipulates these images to search for and highlight abnormalities for further evaluation.

Computerised tomography (CT) uses X-rays to produce cross-sectional slices of the body and contents. A number of two-dimensional X-ray images are taken, rotating around an axis producing several X-ray beams from different angles creating a large amount of radiation. The results are translated by the computer into an image of internal structures in a slice. Some modern scanners can geometrically translate two-dimensional images into three-dimensional (3D), assisting diagnosis through producing a virtual image. CT scans are useful in defining the boundaries of problems such as tumours, abscesses and bleeding, or planning treatments such as radiotherapy. The main lights are dimmed to permit a view of the laser lights required for setting up the image zone. The table moves through a rotational tube to enable imaging of the whole body (Jones and Taylor, 2006).

Magnetic resonance imaging (MRI) uses a magnetic field and radio waves to generate a cross-sectional 3D computer image by manipulating the protons in the body's atoms. As the body is made up predominantly of water it is mainly the hydrogen atoms that are manipulated to create images, making this modality helpful in imaging soft tissue where such atoms are concentrated. The magnetic field arranges the atoms and the application of strong radio waves forces the protons out of position. As they return to their original orientation they give off a signal which is detected by the scanner. This produces an image of the anatomy. MRI is especially good for imaging soft tissue such as brain, heart, abdomen, muscles and joints, blood vessels and breast. Because of the powerful magnetic field used it is important to remove metal objects and jewellery before entering the MRI room. Patients with programmed devices such as pacemakers, implanted defibrillators, cochlea implants, aneurysm clips or previous metallic foreign body eye injuries will not normally be allowed to undergo MRI scanning (Jones and Taylor, 2006). Orthopaedic metal implants such as hip replacement prostheses, internal screws or plates are not usually a problem as they are anchored in place. There is a theoretical risk to the fetus in the first 12 weeks of pregnancy and so MRI scans are usually avoided at this stage. The MRI scanner may cause some patients to feel claustrophobic as they are strapped into position and not allowed to move. The magnet produces a rumbling noise when it is activated. Patients need to be prepared for this and can be offered earplugs to reduce noise irritation.

Nuclear medicine uses radioactive elements known as radioisotopes to target particular organs, or circulatory processes, to diagnose and treat abnormalities. Radioisotopes are specially prepared into pharmacological form for ingesting, injecting, inhaling or implanting. These are then taken up by an organ or cell. They are tracked using a gamma camera, which produces an image of progress and concentration, or through physiological measurements within blood and urine. They may be used to detect foci of infection or tumours, as overactive cells have a greater take-up of radioactive substances. Dosage is important in facilitating diagnostic outcomes without undue radiation effects or suboptimal results. Due to the radioactivity involved they are restricted for use by specially trained personnel. Patients may emit radiation while the substance is in their body, but this usually subsides within a few hours. Longer periods of radioactivity produced by implants mean patients are advised to reduce social contact to avoid exposing other people. This is an important consideration in planning holistic care that encompasses how patients view themselves, their psychosocial well-being in addition to the physical effects (Hart, 2006).

Enhancing imaging

Contrast agents, like air, are used to aid visualisation of structures such as the lungs and the bowel which may be inflated, by air, aiding tissue separation. Contrast media solutions are also used to enhance the quality of images and facilitate diagnosis and treatment. The primary function is to outline structures of the body by attenuating radiation when subjected to an X-ray beam as it progresses to the image intensifier. Contrast is based on salts such as barium sulphate or iodine atoms contained in water-soluble contrast media. Barium sulphate is radiopaque and blocks the X-ray beam, thereby outlining the structure within which it is contained. Such structures are then in contrast to other tissue showing up as white in the resulting image. It is particularly useful for enhancing the gastrointestinal tract (GIT) in barium studies. It is mixed with water to create a suspension with a ratio dependent on the investigation to be performed. The GIT needs to be empty before insertion of the contrast to enable accurate viewing of any filling defects. Fasting and bowel cleansing powders are used in patient preparation to achieve this depending on which test is being undertaken. Side effects of barium sulphate include bloating and constipation necessitating a good fluid intake after the test is completed to help flush the barium out of the body.

Iodine-based contrast media are given intra-arterially, intravenously or inserted into cavities, such as the bladder and uterus, or the biliary and renal tracts. Water-soluble contrast is divided into two main categories: ionic contrasts dissociate into charged particles in solution and non-ionic do not. This has implications for areas of high electrical activity, such as the brain and heart and cellular function, due to ion disturbance. The ratio of iodine atoms to dissolved particles establishes osmolality. Hyperosmolar solutions induce an osmotic pull across cell membranes drawing out water. Low osmolar contrast creates less of an osmotic effect and is therefore safer (Chapman and Nakielny, 2001). Modern contrast agents tend to be low osmolar solutions to reduce the incidence of unwanted effects. The physiological consequences of water shift across the cell membrane include vasodilation, which results in pain, a heat sensation and hypotension. Red blood cells become more rigid as water is drawn out towards the contrast particles. Additive agents include citrate which binds calcium, depressing cardiac contractility and affecting cardiovascular performance. Nurses need to be aware of these consequences in order to monitor and manage patient care during, and following, a procedure involving contrast, in order to distinguish homeostatic consequences of contrast administration from an adverse reaction (Howatson-Jones, 2000).

Contraindications

Iodine-based contrast media are contraindicated for use in individuals with the following conditions:

- Renal/hepatic impairment
- Dehydration
- Sickle cell anaemia
- Heart disease
- Hyperthyroid
- Pregnancy
- History of hypersensitivity
- Asthma triggered by allergy
  (Chapman and Nakielny, 2001, pp. 33–34)

Diabetics who take metformin need to undergo a renal function test prior to the procedure. If this is abnormal then they should not undergo a procedure that uses iodine-based contrast. Where the test is normal, the procedure can go ahead, but metformin should be stopped for 48 hours afterwards and restarted only after a further normal renal function test. This is to ensure that the drug can be adequately excreted; otherwise lactic acidosis may develop. For patients where iodine-based contrast is not suitable an alternative might be to use carbon dioxide (CO_2). This can be injected intra-arterially but needs to be used with caution to avoid cerebral irritation and embolus. It is excreted by blood delivery through the lungs (Jones and Taylor, 2006).

Reactions

There is a high risk of reaction with iodine-based contrast with two mechanisms which can produce reaction symptoms. In the first, activation occurs when there is cross linking between the antigen (in this case iodine from the contrast media) and antibodies present in the plasma that affix to mast and basophil cells triggering a serious immunological reaction. Antibodies are initially formed through prior exposure to iodine, for example, in response to eating seafood which has a high iodine content, so a history of allergy to seafood is significant. The second mechanism is called an anaphylactoid reaction which triggers release of the same mediators through non-immunological means, such as the coagulation, fibrinolytic and kinin-generating systems. It is thought that micro-tissue damage during the procedure such as tears in the endothelial lining of blood vessels stimulates these systems to initiate repair and a chemical response (Morcos, 2005).

Question

Review your understanding of the immune response. How do the coagulation and fibrinolytic and kinin-generating systems operate normally?

A cascade of chemicals is released, including histamine, heparin, chemotactic factor, prostaglandins and leukotrienes (Coico et al., 2003). Their effects are given in Table 7.1.

Vasodilation and increased vasopermeability produce cutaneous effects of erythema, hives and angioedema. Reduction in circulating blood volume and blood pressure occurs as fluid moves out of the vasculature and pools in the peripheral tissues. Bronchoconstriction and simultaneous mucus production lead to dyspnoea and wheezing. It has been found that as anxiety is routed through the hypothalamus of the brain it amplifies effects through the autonomic nervous system, further affecting the respiratory and cardiac centres and triggering the vomiting centre (Lalli, 1980). The crossing of the blood/brain barrier by iodinated contrast also has this effect increasing the risk of respiratory/cardiac arrest. Appropriate emergency drugs should be readily available, including adrenaline (epinephrine); antihistamine,

Table 7.1 Effects of reaction

Substance	Effects
Histamine	Vasodilation, vasopermeability, secretion of mucus, constriction of smooth muscle in the bronchioles
Heparin	Inhibition of coagulation
Chemotactic factor	Influx of eosinophils
Prostaglandins	Vasopermeability, bronchoconstriction, influx of white cells for phagocytosis
Leukotrienes	Vasopermeability, bronchoconstriction, trigger of slow-releasing substance of anaphylaxis prolonging effects

Adapted from Coico et al. (2003).

bronchodilator, atropine to block vagal effects, corticosteroid to reduce continuing effects, intravenous (IV) fluids for blood pressure support and 100% oxygen (Royal College of Radiologists, 2005a). Actual drug choices may vary according to unit protocols. Nursing management strategies include:

- Continual observation and assessment of the patient during procedures
- Providing psychological support to reduce anxiety
- Assessing cardiovascular and respiratory systems and noting any cutaneous effects such as urticaria, hives and angioedema
- Summon medical assistance at first sign of problems
- Commence haemodynamic monitoring, e.g. pulse oximetry, cardiac trace and blood pressure if not already in place
- If blood pressure compromised, lie patient flat and raise legs to increase venous return
- Commence 100% oxygen therapy
- Ensure IV access and have emergency drugs and IV fluids available
- If showing signs of respiratory/cardiac failure, summon crash team and commence CPR as appropriate

Gadolinium is an earth element used as contrast for MRI procedures. It reduces proton relaxation time, enabling clearer images as protons reposition themselves. It is administered intravenously and is excreted through the kidneys but has less of an effect on them than iodinated contrast agents. Side effects include nausea, headache and heat sensation. These are transient and usually pass without requiring medication.

Health and safety

Radiation protection

Radiation poses a danger to people due to its effects on cells. Radiology departments incorporate protective material such as lead in the room structure and doors to

Table 7.2 Recommended dose limits for annual ionising radiation exposure

	Occupational worker	Public
	20 mSv averaging 100 mSv in 5 years	1 mSv
	50 mSv in a single year	
Pregnant	2 mSv abdomen/lower trunk	
	1 mSv equivalent dose to the fetus	–
Eyes	150 mSv	15 mSv
Skin	500 mSv	50 mSv
Hands and feet	500 mSv	–

International Commission for Radiation Protection (2006).

avoid leakage of radiation. Signs and warning lights at the entrances of designated rooms signal their purpose and the potential for exposure. Areas such as CT and MRI restrict entry to the suite through keypad control. The person controlling the exposure is responsible for the safety of people affected. Dose limits are calculated in millisievert (mSv) and based on annual recommended quantities, as provided in Table 7.2 (International Commission for Radiation Protection, 2006). A worker approaching annual dose limits becomes classified and controlled.

Opportunity for the student

Find out what classified and controlled means in relation to working with radiation by visiting http://www.icrp.org.

Protection is based on the principles of justification for exposure, optimisation of protection and limitation of individual dose. For female patients of reproductive age benefits need to outweigh the risks of exposure particularly if there is a possibility that they may be pregnant. Advice from the National Radiation Protection Board (Sharp et al., 1998) (now the Health Protection Agency) and the International Commission on Radiological Protection (2001) suggests that exposure during the 4 weeks from the last menstruation carries a small risk in diagnostic procedures, which increases with higher doses. To be certain of avoiding in utero exposure, women using less reliable forms of contraception need to be within 10 days of the start of their last menstrual period – this rule is applied when a woman is likely to be exposed to significant pelvic radiation. An 18-day rule may be applied for simple X-rays not involving the area between the nipples and the knees. The Royal College of Nursing's (2006) guidance for nurses requires that any female of reproductive age is asked about her pregnancy status and that examinations are planned within 28 days of the onset of the last menstrual period. Where a woman cannot exclude being pregnant advice from the clinician determines the degree of risk and benefit and a serum or urine test may be performed to check for pregnancy. Procedures involving higher doses of radiation, such as CT or barium studies, may need to be postponed.

Regulations set out the duties and actions required to protect the workforce and public (Health and Safety Executive, 1999). Occupational exposure is monitored through a dosimeter worn on the person. Protective clothing includes lead aprons, glasses, thyroid shields and gloves. The eyes and thyroid are particularly sensitive to radiation and hand exposure increases in complex cases. Reproductive areas should be protected by ensuring that the coat, or apron, is of the correct fit and properly fastened. Distance from the X-ray beam reduces exposure dose and should always be maintained where possible. Rooms include radiation shields that either are fixed for standing behind or can be angled to provide additional protection when working near the beam.

Manual handling

Manual handling legislation imposes a duty on the employer of reducing manual handling activity and where this is unavoidable, risk assessing such action. Employees are required to comply with the policies and procedures of the employer (The Manual Handling Operations Regulations, 1992). Amendment to the regulations also demands to consider the physical suitability, knowledge and training, attire, footwear and capability of the employee for carrying out such activity (The Health and Safety – Miscellaneous amendments – Regulations, 2002). It is important that any contraindications in personal capability are communicated to the relevant person. Additional considerations include:

- Assessing necessity and suitability of the activity
- Using equipment provided in accordance with training instructions and correct number of staff
- Ensuring patients are informed and instructed on how to participate in any manual handling exercise

Infection control

Occupational exposure to blood-borne viruses occurs most commonly through percutaneous injuries such as needlestick accidents. A large proportion of these involve nurses (Health Protection Agency, 2005). Injuries occurring intra-operatively often do so because of the complexity of some procedures, whilst postoperatively they tend to result from not complying with safe disposal policies and guidance. Percutaneous injuries should be treated and reported in accordance with local infection control policy guidelines. Many procedures in the radiology department involve body fluids such as urine, faeces and blood. Universal precautions are observed when handling these and care is taken to dispose of sharps in the correct container and manner in accordance with policy guidelines.

To protect patients from microbial infection it is important to clean spillages with the recommended cleaning agents. Patients harbouring known infection are placed at the end of a list, but this should not be at the expense of applying universal precautions to all patients where infection status may be unknown. Strict asepsis is observed for all invasive procedures to avoid the systemic introduction of microbes.

> **Reflection**
>
> Consider the different settings where you have seen infection control precautions applied. Were there any differences, and if so why? What do you conclude are universal precautions and how should these be applied?

Consent

Patients who attend the radiology department may find the environment strange and technical equipment intimidating. They are likely to be anxious about what is going to happen. For this reason consent is obtained by the operative practitioner carrying out the procedure prior to it taking place. Where interventional procedures are involved consent is obtained from the patient before they come to the department. Consent guidance includes:

- Valid consent must be obtained prior to starting a treatment regimen, physical examination or personal care.
- Sufficient information should be given regarding the risks and benefits for the patient to make an informed decision.
- Patients' understanding of what a test is for and why it is being carried out should be ascertained.
- Patients must be kept informed about results and their implications.
  (Department of Health, 2001)

Standards of consent for radiology procedures make a distinction between implied and express consent (Royal College of Radiologists, 2005b). For low-risk procedures, such as a relatively straightforward X-ray, other members of the health care team such as the radiographer will explain the process on behalf of the supervising radiologist. Patient's cooperation with the procedure is deemed to be implied consent. For more complex processes express consent requires a detailed discussion with the patient and verbal or written confirmation of agreement to proceed. For planned invasive procedures, written information should also be supplied in sufficient time for the patient to be able to seek additional information if desired. In an emergency situation the necessity for informed consent is left to the radiologist's judgement. Written consent is essential in procedures that are complex, may impact on the patient's future abilities or are part of a research programme (Royal College of Radiologists, 2005b). Patient autonomy is considered in what patients want to know and their right to give non-informed consent that takes account of them also not wanting to know, but this should be checked with sensitive questioning (see Chapter 2 for questioning techniques). Consent for intimate procedures is sought in an appropriately private setting to allow sensitive explanation and help maintain patient's dignity and privacy in accordance with good practice guidelines (Social Care Institute for Excellence, 2007).

Because of the evolving nature of some procedures as technology and new techniques become available long-term outcomes for these are not as yet known. Gaining consent in such cases requires consideration of:

- What does the procedure involve?
- What are the benefits?
- What is the likelihood of obtaining those benefits?
- Are there alternatives?
- What are the risks?
- Is this risk serious or minor?
- What will happen if the procedure is not undertaken?
  (National Institute for Health and Clinical Excellence (NIHCE), 2003)

Nurses' role

The diversity of the work in the radiology department requires the nurse to coordinate the role across different modalities and a large physical environment. The knowledge and skill base required includes:

- Anatomy and physiology of major body systems
- Radiation protection
- Infection control
- Equipment
- Cannulation
- IV administration
- Resuscitation skills
- Interpersonal skills
  (Royal College of Radiologists; Royal College of Nursing, 2006)

The ability to work without supervision and to use initiative is a key factor. Although a large proportion of patients who attend the radiology department are outpatients, a significant proportion are inpatients who are very ill and it is most often these that the radiology nurse provides care for (Royal College of Radiologists; Royal College of Nursing, 2006). This is particularly relevant as nurses also work on call out of hours. The nurse is part of a multidisciplinary team that includes radiologists, radiographers, technical assistants, office staff and porters, all of whom interlink to provide an efficient, effective and safe service for patients. The nurse's role is to assess patients offering information, support and intervention, as well as assisting with the procedures themselves. For simple screening procedures this involves help in positioning and alleviating anxiety. For interventional procedures the nurse is often the first contact the patient has, making this a primary point of entry into a therapeutic relationship.

Cumulative knowledge

What are the key requirements of a therapeutic relationship and how is this facilitated? Check your answer in Chapter 2.

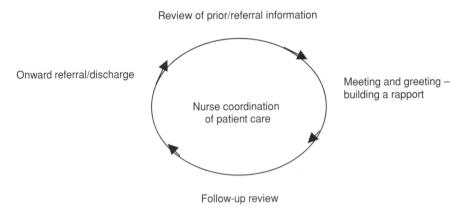

Figure 7.2   Elements of creating trust. [Adapted from Kirschner, 2004.]

The nurse creates a circle of trust with the patient through coordinating care as the patient moves through the department, (Kirschner, 2004) as illustrated in Figure 7.2.

Assessment

Patients attending for outpatient diagnostic procedures are often managed by phone through self-directed contact seeking advice or clarification of preparatory instructions. Patients attending electively for interventional procedures are screened for suitability through pre-assessment techniques (see Chapter 6 on pre-assessment). Routine investigations are completed and reviewed. Patients' understanding of forthcoming procedures and instructions for preparation is established. Specific procedure-related administration can also be arranged, such as infusions for blood clotting or hydration purposes (Jones and Taylor, 2006).

Pre-procedure

The nurse liaises with referring departments and personnel to ensure accurate preparation of the patient (Royal College of Radiologists; Royal College of Nursing, 2006). Patients are assessed by the radiology nurse for suitability on arrival. This is undertaken through interview, scrutiny of notes and detailed handover from ward staff where applicable. Questioning is directed to assessing the psychological and physical state of the patient and allaying anxiety through reassurance. It must be remembered that patients may be disorientated by the unfamiliar environment and reinforcing of information is often required. Patients may be accompanied by friends or family to the department who might also require support. The depth of assessment is determined by the complexity of the procedure and dependency of the patient. Interventional assessment includes the checklist items noted in Figure 7.3.

Patient identifier label	Date:	Radiologist
	Procedure:	Nurse:
	PRE-PROCEDURE CHECKLIST	
Identity		
Consent for procedure		
Pre-medication and time given		
Allergies (in red) (check for seafood)		
Clotting profile	Group and save:	
	Yes/No	
Relevant medical history		
Relevant medication, e.g.		
anticoagulants, aspirin, metformin		
Infections (specify site)		
Pressure areas (state risk score)		
Last menstrual period (where applicable)		
Baseline observations: temperature,		
pulse, respirations, BP, blood sugar if		
applicable		
Signature of nurse:		

Figure 7.3   Interventional procedure checklist

Many centres now use an integrated care plan (ICP) that encompasses multi-professional documentation. Because of the multidisciplinary nature of the team involved in undertaking diagnostic and interventional procedures it is important that relevant information is shared to enable optimum care.

Care planning

Standards of nursing care consider communication and information related to patient autonomy; psychological and physical aspects related to privacy, dignity and comfort; safety issues in terms of infection control, equipment and the environment (RCN, 1993). Planning and documenting care involves considering the patient's current status in terms of difficulties and coping strategies, potential problems and interventions in relation to the above areas (Howatson-Jones, 1999). A team approach should be fostered to promote coordinated care.

Care planning involves prioritisation and decision making. Priorities relate to:

- Informed consent
- Patient condition
- Procedure
- Post-procedure
- Safety issues

Decision making is a dynamic process that occurs as part of continual assessment and reflection-in-action. The critical practitioner processes patient and environmental information from interaction with the patient, inter-professional team and clinical interventions and reacts appropriately. Observation and attentiveness merge with knowledge and experience informing decisions.

Managing pressure sore risk

Interventional procedures are complex and require patients, many of whom already have compromised circulation, to lie immobile for significant periods. Pressure damage begins at the muscle/bone interface and may not become apparent until some time later. X-ray table mattresses are intended to avoid attenuating radiation, which degrades image quality increasing the patient dose, and are not designed for pressure redistribution. Gel mattresses can be used, but these are of varying quality and attenuating factor. Specialist equipment such as bead mattresses that mould to patient shape and hold patient position through application of a vacuum are available but should be used in consultation with radiology staff. These help to increase patient comfort and redistribute pressure but are not pressure reducing. It is important that the length of time on the X-ray table is kept to the minimum required and that pressure area assessments are carried out and communicated with ward staff as part of ongoing care. Pressure monitoring includes establishing the risk score before starting the procedure. Risk factors are posed by:

- Age
- Disease
- Malnourishment
- Mobility
- The procedure – length of time and complexity

Pressure monitoring includes keeping a comfort score that evaluates none, mild, moderate, severe and excruciating discomfort during the procedure to assess coping of the micro-circulation (Mattson Porth, 1994). Strategies to avoid problems include:

- Appropriate manual handling
- Using relevant support devices
- Facilitating minimal repositioning at the onset of discomfort during the procedure

Noting table time, capillary refill time and revised risk score at the end of the procedure informs decisions for ongoing care (Howatson-Jones, 2001). Follow-up skin observations are recommended to assess recovery.

Opportunity for the student

Find out which risk-scoring systems are used in your area. What pressure support systems are available?

Procedural roles

In interventional procedures nurses undertake three roles:

(1) The role of the scrub nurse encompasses acting as assistant to the radiologist and requires a detailed knowledge of procedures and equipment use and function. Preoperative techniques (see Chapter 9) are employed in surgical handwashing, gowning and gloving and aseptic preparation of the equipment trolley and patient's sterile field. Theatre attire is worn over radiation-protective clothing. The nurse prepares the equipment and monitors its condition during the procedure, keeping order on the trolley and patient's sterile field to avoid accidental contamination and loss. Drugs are checked, labelled and identified for the radiologist and administration noted. The nurse anticipates the progress of the procedure in order to have necessary equipment ready, helping to maintain a minimal screening and table time. At the end of the procedure all equipment and sharps are accounted for and disposed of into the appropriate container. Descrubbing follows the procedure outlined in Chapter 9.

(2) The circulating nurse assists the scrub nurse in surgical preparation and setting up the equipment trolley by passing required items at the start of and during the procedure. A record is kept of items and drugs used. This nurse introduces him/herself and prepares the patient through offering reassurance and explanation of activities, helping with positioning and attaching monitoring devices. Throughout the procedure the circulating nurse maintains patient contact, offering frequent reassurance and support and assessing physiological status through haemodynamic and respiratory monitoring. Any abnormalities are immediately reported to the radiologist and remedial measures taken. Pain relief may be administered as requested and prescribed by the radiologist. The nurse completes intra-operative documentation and notes procedural end time and any items permanently placed, such as a stent. The patient is assisted back into their bed and observations of the wound and vital signs undertaken.

(3) The recovery nurse's role is often an extension of the circulating nurse role. Where it is undertaken by another member of the team a careful and thorough handover of procedural progress and patient condition is required. The patient is moved to a quiet recovery area away from the main waiting zones and monitoring of vital signs, puncture wound and conscious status, where applicable, continue until the patient is deemed stable and ready to return to the ward. The recovery process is documented and a handover and follow-up instructions are given to the ward nurse.

Opportunity for the student

Look at the monitoring equipment used. What does it do and what is the purpose in using it? How do you interpret displayed readings?

Communication and advocacy

Radiology work utilises a list system which creates pressure for continuity as delay may cause cancellation of following procedures. Comfort is minimal and some interventions may induce pain. Patient advocacy in such an environment is a crucial part of the nursing role as the coordinator of care. The nurse liaises within and outside the department and provides specialist instruction. This requires skill in inter-professional communication and teamworking.

Cumulative knowledge

What are some likely advocacy opportunities that might arise in the radiology department? How might you advocate for patients?

Check your answer by referring back to the communication strategies in Chapter 2.

Health education and health promotion

Patients attend for procedures that are related to a wide variety of conditions and diseases. The nurse is able to explain the procedure, but also relates its purpose to understanding disease mechanisms providing information on the disease process. Patients' understanding of their condition is gauged and augmented as required. Aftercare advice provides health promotion opportunities in considering lifestyle changes as part of procedural recovery and future disease management.

Opportunities for the student

Observe which health promotion strategies are used and why. How do they link to current National Service Frameworks (NSFs) used in the UK?

Developments in the nursing role

The role of the imaging nurse has advanced considerably beyond setting up equipment for procedures to taking an active part. Further areas that are currently being explored include:

- Pre-assessment
- Evaluation of procedural requests
- Minor procedures
- Patient discharge
- Liaison with other agencies
- Establishment of a modern matron role
  (Royal College of Radiologists; Royal College of Nursing, 2006)

In addition, studies have been undertaken into nurses performing diagnostic angiography with favourable results (Morgan et al., 2001). This advanced role is complemented by advanced study at masters degree level. With the need to deliver an 18-week Patient Pathway Programme for imaging (National Imaging Board, 2007) that reduces the waiting time from referral to treatment to 18 weeks, all staff are required to develop their roles across traditional boundaries to increase capacity and a seamless service for patients.

Management of equipment

Radiological procedures select from a large portfolio of expensive equipment. It is important to maintain regularity of supply and availability of disposable items to ensure procedures can be undertaken at the correct time. Stock rotation, including drugs, is necessary to avoid expensive wastage due to exceeding expiry dates. Many items are now available on consignment order of sale when items are used or returned within a specified time frame. Correct storage of specialist disposable stock avoids damage. Sterile equipment is removed from packaging only when actually requested during a procedure and is checked for any damage prior to use. Where damage is found the item is kept for return to the supplier. Regular checking of resuscitation and monitoring equipment is necessary to ensure accurate working order.

Part 2: Diagnostic procedures

Patient preparation

Explanation and reassurance are the main requirements of patient preparation. The nurse assembles the relevant equipment. For intimate procedures an appropriate nurse also acts as a chaperone if required.

General diagnostic procedures involving nursing input:

- *Venogram* – Although commonly undertaken in the past, new Doppler techniques have largely made this procedure redundant. However, it is still used for renal patients to check arteriovenous fistulae and is called a fistulogram. Contrast is injected to demonstrate the patency of the local venous system and outline any defects.
  (1) Cannulation equipment and contrast are prepared.
  (2) The appropriate vein is cannulated and contrast injected.
  (3) Pressure is applied on removal of the cannula to achieve haemostasis.
- *Herniogram* – Contrast is injected into the abdominal cavity to outline abdominal contents.
  (1) Local anaesthetic is given.

(2) Contrast is injected through a long needle that punctures the abdominal wall and abdominal X-rays taken whilst changing position of the patient.

(3) Aftercare requires the application of a sticking plaster and short period of observation for any ill effects.

- *Micturating cystogram* – It demonstrates bladder function and ureteral reflux. This procedure is mainly undertaken in paediatric patients.

  (1) The patient is usually catheterised by the nurse (an advanced practice skill with this age group) and the bladder filled with contrast by the radiologist.

  (2) The catheter is removed and patients empty their bladder under X-ray visualisation.

- *Hysterosalpingogram* – Due to the intimacy of this procedure the staff involved will usually be female, including the radiologist. Contrast is injected under pressure into the cervix and uterus to demonstrate patency and spillage from the fallopian tubes and any filling defects in the uterus, such as fibroids. X-ray screening tracks the flow of contrast.

  (1) Menstrual dates are checked.

  (2) A speculum is inserted and the cervix visualised and contrast injected under pressure through a soft, flexible small-gauge catheter.

  (3) Aftercare includes advising the patient of blood spotting, infective discharge and other signs of infection, e.g. pyrexia.

- *Barium studies* – These include barium swallow and barium meal which the patient swallows and barium enema with barium introduced through an enema tube followed by inflation of the bowel with air. X-rays are taken to follow the flow of barium with the patient changing position.

  (1) Nurses may assist with positioning and hygiene needs if required, but these procedures form only a small part of the nurse's role.

Mammography

Women are routinely screened every 3 years between the ages of 47 and 73 years as part of the National Breast Screening Programme in the UK to detect abnormalities such as breast cancer. Younger women are screened only if there is a high-risk family history.

Where an abnormality is detected a triple assessment is undertaken; this also applies to men who may also present with breast abnormalities. Triple assessment involves a physical examination, mammography and biopsy if appropriate. Biopsies may be undertaken under ultrasound or X-ray control and may take a few cells and/or a core of tissue. A fine-needle aspiration biopsy involves removing some of the cells from the abnormal area with a needle and syringe. A core biopsy involves using a tru-cut needle to remove a core of tissue under local anaesthetic for analysis. Women attending for screening are naturally very apprehensive of the potential diagnosis and require considerable psychological support. The nurse is essential in offering such support and providing distraction techniques and assistance during biopsy procedures.

Scenario

Mrs Green is a civil servant. She is Caucasian, 42 years old and married with two teenage children. She has recently taken advantage of a local scheme that allows her to have a mammogram for a nominal fee as she is aged within the 40–50 band. She has been called back to the National Health Services clinic for further tests because of abnormalities on the mammogram. She attends the breast clinic with her husband and is naturally very anxious. She undergoes a triple assessment. This includes a physical examination and further mammograms. An impalpable mass is found on these films requiring her to undergo an X-ray-guided core biopsy which is sent to the laboratory for analysis.

(1) Which laboratory will the sample be sent to and what are the scientists looking for?
(2) What are the main issues and your priorities in this situation?
(3) What ethical issues might arise?

Interventional procedures

Patient preparation:

- Ensure written consent is obtained.
- Ensure patient is not on anticoagulants. If on a drug with a short half-life then this would need to be stopped 1 day before the procedure; if on a longer acting variety then this would need to be stopped 4 days before. If taking aspirin, the reason for taking it needs to be checked as the benefits may outweigh the risk of having less platelets available for clotting.
- Check for allergies such as to seafood.
- Clotting profile that may or may not include group and save. Clotting is necessary to ensure that haemostasis can be achieved where the integrity of tissue is breached, to avoid haemorrhage.
- Depending on whether any sedative drugs are likely to be used, diet may continue up to 4 hours pre-procedure and then only fluids are taken. Some procedures require the patient to be nil by mouth, particularly if sedation is likely to be involved. Because of the risk of haemorrhage patients undergoing major interventional procedures need to be prepared as for theatre (see Chapter 9).
- Pre-medication is used less commonly as most procedures involve local anaesthetic, but it may be given if the patient is very anxious. Because many interventional procedures require the patient to lie still, anxiety can be a problem. Sedative pre-medication may be offered to aid patient comfort during the procedure (Royal College of Radiologists, 2003).
- IV access is required for complicated procedures, such as arterial embolisation and stent insertion, to allow administration of analgesia as well as sedation. Cooperative protocols between radiology and anaesthetic departments ensure that appropriate personnel are involved in the administration of sedation for radiological procedures (Royal College of Radiologists, 2003).

- Inform the radiologist if the patient takes metformin or their blood glucose is high.
- For reproductive females check the date of the last menstrual period.
- Baseline observations of temperature, pulse, respiratory rate and blood pressure. A raised blood pressure will increase the risk of post-procedural haemorrhage and so the radiologist should be notified for a decision on continuation.
- Preoperative checklist and escort. The radiology nurse needs information regarding the patient so that appropriate care can be given.

General interventional procedures

- *Angiography* – The introduction of contrast into an artery helps identify narrowing or other defects.
  (1) Local anaesthetic is injected around the femoral artery which is then punctured. This is the safest site of entry as it is easy to compress against bone for haemostasis at the end.
  (2) A guide wire directs catheter placement, which is followed by contrast injection and image acquisition.
  (3) Pressure is applied for 10 min following removal.
  MRI has made the necessity for this invasive procedure less common as enhanced magnetic resonance angiography (MRA) has advanced using manipulation of visual planes to produce an image of the arteries. CT is also beginning to be employed to produce a six-slice contrast-enhanced image that will also avoid the invasiveness of traditional angiography.
- *Thrombolysis* – This procedure is now undertaken more rarely as other treatment methods have advanced. The procedure involves insertion of a clot-dissolving agent called recombinant tissue plasminogen activator (r-TPA) that breaks up the fibrin structure of the clot. It is given by initial bolus through the catheter which is then connected to a continuous infusion that needs to be shielded from light. The treatment may last up to 48 hours.
  (1) Contraindications for the procedure include recent haemorrhagic problems or surgery.
  (2) Aftercare is undertaken in a high-dependency area to ensure close monitoring due to the high risk of haemorrhage.
- *Angioplasty* – Treatment of narrowing in an artery with a balloon that is inflated and flattens the obstruction along the arterial wall.
- *Endovascular aneurysm repair* – This procedure uses a multidisciplinary approach involving the theatre, surgical and radiological team. The patient is often given a spinal anaesthetic (see Chapter 9 for explanation of this type of anaesthetic) and the surgical team performs a cut down to both femoral arteries for direct visualisation. The radiologist inserts a stent graft which extends into the aorta to protect the arterial wall from further pressure.
- *Stenting* – Insertion of a metal corrugated or plastic cylindrical tube delivered via a balloon to maintain patency of a vessel. Used for persistent arterial narrowing where angioplasty has failed or for carcinoma and strictures, e.g. biliary tract and colon.

- *Embolisation* – It involves deliberate occlusion of a vessel to terminate blood flow. It may be arterial to induce necrosis of an area, e.g. uterine fibroids, liver metastases, or venous to reduce engorgement and pain, e.g. ovarian or testicular varicies (a weakness and bulging in the particular vein). Embolisation may also be used as an emergency measure to stem post-partum haemorrhage after childbirth where the bleeding site is difficult to ascertain surgically.
  (1) Analgesia is required for arterial interventions undertaken to produce necrosis as these are very painful when ischaemia begins.
  (2) Chemotherapy prescription may be necessary for liver malignancy as this drug is placed and then sealed in by the embolisation.
  (3) Antibiotics may be used in arterial procedures as prophylaxis against infection according to radiologist choice.
  (4) Venous embolisation does not require any specific preparation or analgesia.
- *Insertion of caval filter* – This is applied to the inferior vena cava to trap emboli travelling from the deep veins to the pulmonary system reducing the risk of pulmonary embolism where there are problems with the use of anticoagulants. The patient is able to go home after 1–2 hours.
- *Needle biopsies* – These are undertaken for locating and diagnosing tumours, such as renal, liver, prostate and breast, or cell types, e.g. renal for the presence of glomeruli.
- *Aspiration* – This is undertaken for fluid collections usually under ultrasound or CT control, e.g. abdominal and pelvic.
- *Percutaneous drainage* – Where normal flow has been blocked a drain may be inserted under imaging control, e.g. in the biliary or renal tract which is blocked by stones or tumours.
- *Insertion of gastrostomy tube* – Where there are upper gastrointestinal or other problems and endoscopic placement has failed, direct percutaneous access through the stomach wall is obtained under imaging control and the tube inserted. This procedure is commonly undertaken with patients who have motor neurone disease (MND) and who, therefore, may have difficulty communicating. It is vital that whatever methods of communication that the patient normally uses are employed to aid explanation and reduce anxiety during the procedure. These may include alphabet boards for example. Patients need to have a nasogastric tube in place before attendance for this procedure.

Biliary – The hepatic duct is punctured and a catheter is placed to allow the system to decompress for a few days by drainage before being followed with a stent insertion. Patient preparation includes:
(1) Nil by mouth 4 hours preoperatively in case of complications requiring surgery
(2) Broad spectrum antibiotics 12 hours pre- and post-procedure
(3) IV access for analgesia and sedation as this is a very painful procedure
Renal – The pelvis of the kidney is punctured and a pigtail nephrostomy drainage tube placed to decompress the kidney, saving the potential of further tissue damage caused by obstruction. The tube locks into position when the pigtail is formed at the end. Sometimes it may be possible to extend a guide wire down through

the ureter at the time of trying to place a nephrostomy tube and insert a stent instead that traverses from the kidney to the bladder, avoiding the drainage tube which is awkward and uncomfortable.

Patient aftercare following interventional procedures:

General

- Quarter hourly blood pressure, pulse and puncture site observations for 4 hours. These intervals should *not* be expanded as the greatest risk of haemorrhage is during the first 4 hours.
- Bed rest as specified by the interventional practitioner. Usually 24 hours for complex arterial or other potentially haemorrhagic procedures.
- May resume normal diet.

Embolisation

- Embolisation syndrome – Due to an ischaemia-induced inflammatory response patients may complain of flu-like symptoms of low-grade pyrexia and general malaise 24 hours after the procedure. These last about 48 hours. High pyrexia is indicative of infection and should *always* be reported.
- Analgesia – It is required regularly for arterial embolisation pain.

Thrombolysis, angioplasty, stenting, biopsy

- Check for retention of normal function.
- Thrombolysis patients can only have oral fluids until the infusion is complete.

Gastrostomy

- The tube may be used 4 hours post-procedure.
- Flushing – keep the line patent with regular flushing of sterile water.

Complications

Vascular (at the puncture site)

- Haemorrhage – due to poor plug formation
- Thrombosis – due to clot formation
- Haematoma – due to undetected bleeding
- Pseudoaneurysm – weakening of the arterial wall due to equipment use
- Infection
- Neural damage as nerve is sited near the artery
- Arteriovenous fistula – formed by initial puncture

Systemic

- Renal impairment due to contrast-induced disruption of kidney function
- Septicaemia – due to introduction of infection into bloodstream
- Tumour overgrowth/ingrowth of stenting device

Scenario

Mrs Green, 42, re-attends from the day surgery unit for localisation of impalpable breast lump, which involves inserting a wire guide under X-ray control mammograms to guide the surgeon to the area to be removed. She is very nervous. She will go straight to theatre after this.

(1) What issues might you need to plan for?

Summary

Radiological nursing has been demonstrated as encompassing a large range of procedures and knowledge. The nursing role has been perceived in the context of a multidisciplinary team that makes this a public arena in which to provide nursing care requiring good advocacy skills. Opportunities for the student have been highlighted in considering pressure area risk scoring systems, monitoring equipment and health promotion strategies in this area. Reflection on the implications of universal precautions enables students to critically add to their experience of infection control in diverse environments.

Acknowledgement

The author acknowledges the helpful discussion and reading of the chapter for accuracy by Rebecca Clark, Matron for Radiological Sciences and Clinical Governance, East Kent Hospitals Trust.

Glossary of terms

Anaphylactoid
Elements of the immune response but reached through other physiological pathways

Anaphylaxis
Serious immune response that causes cardiovascular and respiratory collapse

Angioplasty
Dilating a blocked artery by insertion and inflation of a balloon

Arteriogram
X-ray examination of the arterial system

Attenuation
Degree of absorption of radiation

Bronchoconstriction
Narrowing of the bronchioles

Contrast
Agent that enhances imaging

Cutaneous
Of the skin and underlying tissue

Embolisation
Deliberate occlusion of a vessel

Haemodynamic
Function of blood circulation

Haemotoma
Blood clot under the skin

Half-life
Time for plasma concentration of the drug to decrease by half

Homeostasis
Ability to maintain equilibrium within the body

Ionic
Charged particles in solution

Osmolality
Concentration of a solution

Stent
Metal or plastic tube inserted to keep a vessel patent

Thrombosis
Blood clot in a blood vessel

Urticaria
Itchy rash

Vasodilation
Relaxation of blood vessels

Vasopermeability
Opening of spaces in the blood vessel walls

Websites

www.goingfora.com
http://www.icrp.org

References

Chapman, S. and Nakielny, R. (2001) *A Guide to Radiological Procedures*, 4th ed. Edinburgh: Saunders.

Coico, R., Sunshine, G. and Benjamini, E. (2003) *Immunology: A Short Course*, 5th ed. Chichester: John Wiley and Sons Ltd.

Department of Health (2001) *Reference Guide to Consent for Examination or Treatment* [online]. Available from: http://www.dh.gov.uk/assetRoot/04/01/90/79/04019079.pdf (accessed 1 July 2006).

Hart, S. (2006) Ionising radiation: promoting safety for patients, visitors and staff. *Nursing Standard 20* (47), pp. 47–57.

Health and Safety Executive (1999) *The Ionizing Radiations Regulations 1999 No: 3232* [online]. Available from: http://www.legislation.hmso.gov.uk/si/si1999/19993232.htm (accessed 16 August 2006).

Health Protection Agency (2005) Eye of the Needle: Surveillance of Significant Occupational Exposure to Bloodborne Viruses in Healthcare Workers. Center for Infections; England, Wales and Northern Ireland Seven Year Report [online]. Available from: http://www.hpa?q=eye+of+the+needle&sa.x=7&sa.y=9 (accessed 14 August 2006).

Howatson-Jones, I.L. (2000) Adverse reactions to contrast media. *Professional Nurse 15*(12), pp. 771–774.

Howatson-Jones, I.L. (2001) Relieving the pressure in the radiology department. *British Journal of Nursing 10*(4), pp. 219–228.

Howatson-Jones, L. (1999) Arterial embolisation of uterine fibroids. *Nursing Standard 13*(45), pp. 41–45.

International Commission on Radiological Protection (2001) *Radiation and Your Patient: A Guide for Medical Practitioners. ICRP Supporting Guidance 2* [online]. Available from: http://www.sciencedirect.com/science (accessed 9 August 2006).

International Commission on Radiological Protection (2006) ICRP SG5: analysis of the criteria used by the International Commission on Radiological Protection to justify the setting of numerical protection value levels. *Annals of the ICRP 36*(4), pp. 1–78 [online]. Available from: http://www.sciencedirect.com/science/journal/01466453 (accessed 10 October 2007).

Jones, S. and Taylor, E.J. (2006) *Imaging for Nurses*. Oxford: Blackwell Publishing.

Kirschner R. (2004) Creating a circle of trust. *Journal of Radiology Nursing 23*(2), p. 52 [online]. Available from: http://www.sciencedirect.com/science (accessed 10 January 2006).

Lalli, A.F. (1980) Contrast media reactions: data analysis and hypotheses. *Radiology 134*(1), pp. 1–12.

Mattson Porth, C. (1994) *Pathophysiology, Concepts of Altered Health States*, 4th ed. Philadelphia: JB Lippencott.

Morcos, S.K. (2005) Acute serious and fatal reactions to contrast media: our current understanding. *The British Journal of Radiology 78*, pp. 686–693.

Morgan, R., Wallis, L. and Belli, A.-M. (2001) Diagnostic angiography performed by nurses. *The British Journal of Radiology 74*, pp. 648–650.

National Imaging Board (2007) *Delivery of the 18 Week Patient Pathway and Beyond: A Strategy for Imaging Workforce National Imaging Board Strategy* [online]. Available from: http://www.18weeks.nhs.uk/public/default.aspx?main=true&load=ArticleViewer&ArticleId=562 (accessed 24 September 2007).

National Institute for Health and Clinical Excellence (NIHCE) (2003) *Consent – Procedures for Which the Benefits and Risks are Uncertain*. London: National Institute for Health and Clinical Excellence.

Royal College of Nursing (RCN) (1993) *Radiology Nursing: Standards of Care*. London: Royal College of Nursing.

Royal College of Nursing (RCN) (2006) *Best Practice Guidance on Pregnancy Testing Prior to Diagnostic Imaging*. London: Royal College of Nursing.

Royal College of Radiologists (RCR) (2003) *Safe sedation, analgesia and anaesthesia within the Radiology Department* [online]. Available from: http://www.rcr.ac.uk/index.asp?PageID=310&PublicationID=186#Anchor-Executive-21683 (accessed 10 October 2007).

Royal College of Radiologists (RCR) (2005a) *Standards for Iodinated Intravascular Contrast Agent Administration to Adult Patients*. London: Royal College of Radiologists.

Royal College of Radiologists (RCR) (2005b) *Standards for Patient Consent Particular to Radiology*. London: Royal College of Radiologists.

Royal College of Radiologists; The Royal College of Nursing (2006) *Guidelines for Nursing Care in Interventional Radiology*. London: Royal College of Radiologists.

Sharp, C., Shrimpton, J.A. and Bury, R.F. (1998) *Diagnostic Medical Exposures. Advice on Exposure to Ionizing Radiation During Pregnancy* [online]. Oxon: National Radiation Protection Board. Available from: http://www.hpa.org.uk/radiation/publications/misc_publications/advice_during_pregnancy.htm (accessed 14 August 2006).

Social Care Institute for Excellence (2007) *Practice Guide 09. Dignity in Care* [online]. Available from: http://www.scie.org.uk/publications/practiceguides/practiceguide09/index.asp (accessed 2 October 2007).

The Health and Safety (Miscellaneous Amendments) Regulations (2002) *Statutory Instrument 2002 No: 2174* [online]. Available from: http://www.opsi.gov.uk/si/si2002/20022174.htm (accessed 16 August 2006).

The Manual Handling Regulations (1992) *Statutory Instrument 1992 No 2793* [online]. Available from: http://www.opsi.gov.uk/si/si1992/Uksi_19922793_en_1.htm (accessed 16 August 2006).

Watkinson, A.F., Francis, I.S., Torrie, P. and Platts, A.D. (2002) The role of anaesthesia in interventional radiology. *The British Journal of Radiology 75*, pp. 105–106.

Chapter 8

Endoscopy nursing

Lioba Howatson-Jones

Learning objectives

(1) Identify the role of the nurse in preparing and supporting the patient for endoscopy
(2) Demonstrate knowledge of health and safety good practice in this area
(3) Describe a variety of key endoscopic procedures
(4) Identify appropriate preparation and aftercare
(5) Describe potential complications and management strategies
(6) Consider future developments in the nursing role

Introduction

Definition

Endoscopy involves visualising the inside of body tracts for diagnosis and treatment, either through direct means, or in association with radiological imaging modalities.

The NHS Plan (Department of Health (DH), 2000a) and improvement plan (DH, 2004) call for health professionals to develop techniques that reduce the need for hospital-based interventions through the harnessing of new technologies. The NHS

Cancer Plan (DH, 2000b) requires earlier diagnosis for cancer patients by establishing screening programmes, increasing the use of endoscopy services through, for example, the bowel screening programme. Significant progress is being made in modernising and expanding diagnostic facilities such as endoscopy (National Audit Office, 2005). Such legislative and economic trends are the impetus behind the rising profile of endoscopic interventions. Endoscopic techniques have advanced rapidly with new imaging modalities emerging, particularly in the digital sphere. Innovations in flexible endoscopic instrumentation make it possible for increasingly complex diagnostic and therapeutic uses. Possibilities for biopsy, ligation and the resection of polyps have promoted cooperation with other services, such as radiology, to reduce the need for surgery. Virtual colonoscopy and spectroscopy for analysing tissue is becoming a reality, adding another dimension to diagnosis. Such developments have helped reduce the need for hospitalisation but necessitate a higher degree of collaboration between departments, services and with patients, to ensure they are able to self-care before and after procedures. Nursing knowledge correspondingly needs to keep pace with these changes in order to provide optimum patient care and health education. The endoscopy service can be undertaken in primary care settings as well as provide for outpatients and inpatients in the hospital environment.

This chapter begins by considering equipment relating to the science of endoscopic visualisation explaining the capturing of images through light transmission, and exploring developing modalities. Health and safety are related to care of endoscopic equipment and decontamination as part of infection control. It is not the intention of the text to provide a comprehensive list of all endoscopic procedures, but rather it describes the nursing role in assessment, care aspects and management strategies of selected procedures that are undertaken in the endoscopy environment. It does not include other endoscopic procedures that might be undertaken in the surgical field of practice. Opportunities for the student in the endoscopy environment are highlighted. Department infrastructure makes this a rather public arena in which to carry out assessment and intimate examinations, requiring good communication and advocacy skills and providing opportunities for the student to develop these further. Finally, the developing role of the nurse endoscopist and future progression are explored.

The science of endoscopic visualisation instrumentation

An endoscope is a steerable, flexible tube with multiple channels for additional instrumentation that connects to a light source, using xenon and fibre optic technology to illuminate internal structures with intense light, allowing examination through visualisation. Xenon technology provides intense illumination by emitting short pulse light across a wide spectrum helping to provide realistic colour of tissue. Electrical energy is stored in a capacitor and, when activated, ionises the xenon gas in a sealed tube discharging energy. This is converted into optical energy in the lamp (Jacobson and Katzman, 2001). The cabling carries the light and returns images for viewing by the operator. Digital video camera equipment is used to capture, edit and store images to monitor progress of the procedure and record animated and still images of particular interest. Recent technological developments now allow images to be shown in high-definition format through charge-coupled devices placed at the tip of the endoscope (Radford, 2005). Alternatively, endoscopic ultrasonography uses high-frequency sound waves to outline internal structures by detecting the different signals produced and reflected back, which are translated into an image (Ogilvie et al., 2002).

Developing complementary modalities includes the introduction of virtual imaging that is non-invasive and particularly useful in groups at high risk of bleeding. One such procedure is virtual colonoscopy, which visualises the colon by using computerised tomography (CT) (see Chapter 7 for how this works) to produce thin pictured slices of the colon which are manipulated into two- and three-dimensional images by the computer. This is called CT colonography. The images are then interpreted by a radiologist. Additional preparation and training are recommended to increase the accuracy of such interpretation (Macari and Bini, 2005). Patient preparation is essential to ensure the bowel is empty so that faecal matter does not obscure lesions, such as polyps. Some recommend the use of additional intravenous contrast because this enhances the visibility of polyps, but the advantages of this method need to be tempered with the potential for side effects and the risk of a contrast-mediated reaction. New diagnostic techniques are evolving in the use of light-scattering spectroscopy and optical coherence tomography. These beam light waves into suspect tissue giving a reading that is converted into graph form, or which provides a depth image 'similar to a pathology slide' (Glenn, 2001, p. 272). These are particularly useful for diagnosing cancers.

Health and safety

An endoscope comprises a flexible body with a combined air, water and suction channel and adjunct instrument channel for use of accessories such as biopsy forceps, snares and stone removal baskets, as well as cleaning equipment (Radford, 2005). Air is required to separate structures by inflation enabling viewing, whilst water and suction facilitate the removal of obscuring matter. Associated equipment includes the light feed cabling and camera.

Endoscopes are costly instruments and are stored in a lockable facility to avoid loss or interference. They require special care and attention in handling and, because of their delicacy, are stored in vertical racks to avoid damage to the fibre optic component and cabling. Regular maintenance schedules, through medical engineering departments and equipment manufacturers, ensure readiness for use and avoidance of malfunction during procedures that could adversely affect the patient (Radford, 2005). The equipment is inspected before, during and after use to ensure no visual defects are evident, and that accessory equipment such as light sources and combined water, air and suction channels are working.

Body fluids carry the risk of transferring pathogens and need to be eliminated from instrumentation through cleaning and disinfection processes. Decontamination involves a combination of cleaning, disinfecting and sterilising to render a reusable item safe for further use with patients, and by staff, minimising the risk of transmission of infectious agents (DH, 2003). Because of their delicacy flexible endoscopes cannot be placed in an autoclave, or steam steriliser. Cleaning, therefore, is achieved through washing and application of chemical disinfectants that can cause irritation to the user. Prior to cleaning leak tests are performed to avoid incurring damage through submersion in fluid. Where damage is detected the endoscope is removed from service, cleaned according to manufacturer instruction and sent for repair (Association of Perioperative Registered Nurses, 2003). The Medicines and Healthcare products Regulatory Agency (MHRA) (2006) recommends that the endoscope and accessories are manually cleaned prior to processing with disinfectant and that all channels should be flushed, even if they were not used during the procedure. The advent of automated washers has helped to reduce exposure of staff to chemicals, but these need to be used correctly to ensure no recontamination occurs through, for example, inadequately filtering and sterilising the rinse water (Radford, 2005). It is recommended that decontamination is carried out at the beginning of a list, between patients and at the end of the working day by staff trained in these techniques, and undertaken in specialist rooms. Cleaning needs to include an enzymatic detergent and brushing with a single-use brush (British Society of Gastroenterology Working Party Report, 2003). Quality assurance audits, which look at the adequacy of rinse water filtration and disinfection of cleaning processes are undertaken to ensure consistency and adherence to guidelines. These audits involve random culture sampling of endoscopes; positive results require action by management (Ogilvie et al., 2002).

The emergence of variant Creuzfeldt Jacob disease (vCJD) has led to further modification of procedures. The risk of transmitting infectious prions (proteins) from an infected patient via instrument use to another, has necessitated replacing some reusable equipment with single-use items because cleaning does not totally remove, or deactivate, such material. This is particularly relevant in neuroendoscopy which involves high-risk nerve tissue where it is recommended that single-use accessories are always used (National Institute for Health and Clinical Excellence (NIHCE), 2006). Any procedure that breaches gut mucosa, such as a gastrointestinal biopsy which brings material through a working channel, is deemed invasive. Of significance here is the potential exposure to lymphoid tissue. In 'at risk' patients disposable biopsy forceps are used and the endoscope is quarantined (taken out of service). 'High-risk' groups include those with haemophilia, as well as others exhibiting symptoms of vCJD (British Society of Gastroenterology Decontamination Working Group, 2005a).

Opportunity for the student

What are the decontamination procedures in your unit? Which equipment is reused and what is single use? What is the reasoning behind this? (Refer to Chapter 7 for discussion on universal precautions.)

Nursing role

The role of the nurse is to work independently, as well as collaborate with other members of the health care team in making care decisions. Key aspects of the role include:

- Establishing nursing priorities through assessment and nursing diagnosis that identify patient-focused outcomes and plan care accordingly
- Practicing ethical decision making to ensure safe and effective patient care
- Assisting the endoscopist in diagnostic and interventional procedures
- Administering pharmacological and therapeutic treatment regimes
- Undertaking monitoring and diagnostic activity as required by the endoscopist
- Responding to emergency situations through recognition of changes in patient health status and implementing support mechanisms
- Documenting patient monitoring results ensuring continuity of care
- Managing aftercare and follow-up
- Providing health education and health promotion to patients and significant others
- Participating in educational activities for their own continuing professional development and in the teaching and mentoring of others
  (Adapted from Society of Gastroenterology Nurses and Associates (SGNA), 2005.)

The nursing role in relation to patient care is directed to establishing a therapeutic relationship by welcoming patients and sharing information, while assessing compliance with preparatory instructions and the patients' current health status. Assessment of the patient is undertaken to determine relevant medical and personal history, and their physical and psychological ability to undergo the proposed procedures and tolerate any potential drug therapy.

Particular attention is given to identifying patient concerns and anxieties. Explanation helps promote patient involvement in care planning and decision making, potentially minimising distress, provided choices are offered with regard to the depth of description and the use of sedation, where appropriate. Choice of attire when complete undress is not required also helps a patient to maintain a sense of independence and dignity (Social Care Institute for Excellence, 2007). Knowledge of individual patient need from the start enables planning post-procedure care that takes account of patient preference in the interventions proposed, whilst also considering relevant health promotion strategies. Due to the short time from assessment to procedure, the nurse plays a crucial role in the informing element of consent. This occurs through preparatory explanations helping patients to assimilate complete accounts of the risks and benefits of the procedure given by the endoscopist. Ethical practice dictates that patients make autonomous decisions about what happens to them, whilst there is a legal requirement that the endoscopist discusses alternatives to the procedure proposed and the management of potential complications (Breier-Mackie, 2005). The nurse's involvement ensures continuing monitoring of patient choice during the procedure and potential for advocating where a patient might change their mind.

Cumulative knowledge

What are the ethical and legal requirements for gaining informed consent? How can patients become empowered? (Return to Chapter 2 on communication to check your answer.)

Documentation

Documentation is fundamental to the nursing process of planning care that is individual to the patient and includes assessment, identified goals, planned interventions, implementation and evaluation. It follows patient progression through the phases of pre-procedure, procedure and post-procedure (SGNA, 2003). Table 8.1 identifies some of the key areas that are included.

Table 8.1 Core requirements of procedural documentation based on SGNA (2003) guidelines

Pre-procedure	Procedure	Post-procedure
Verification of patient identity and details	Verification of procedure and patient	Time entering recovery phase and verification of patient details
Health assessment questionnaire including compliance with preparatory instructions	Type of procedure and therapeutic processes undertaken including equipment used	Condition of patient and procedural instruction for continuing aftercare
Baseline observations of temperature, pulse, respirations, blood pressure, oxygenation, consciousness/mental state	Monitoring observations of pulse, respirations, blood pressure, oxygenation, consciousness and pain	Post-procedural observations of pulse, respirations, blood pressure, oxygenation, consciousness and pain
Medication	Drug and fluid administration and effect	Drug and fluid administration and effect
Allergies	Adverse reactions	Unusual events
Relevant clinical investigation results	Samples taken during the examination	Identify how the patient will obtain results
Understanding of procedure and health educational needs	Time procedure commenced and completed	Adherence to discharge criteria
Patient concerns	Condition of the patient at completion of the procedure	Post-procedural informing including patient concerns, health education and health promotion
Follow-up support	Handover and follow-up instructions	Escort/home carer instruction, onward referral details
Identity of completing health professional	Identity of all attending health personnel	Identity of completing health professional

---

Checkpoint

How do the core requirements for documentation fit with the nursing process framework of care planning?

Preparing for endoscopic procedures

It is recommended that, as a minimum, a registered nurse is available in each of the areas of pre-procedure, the endoscopy room and recovery. This is of particular importance where intravenous sedation is used. Where a procedure is more complex additional staff are required, although some of these may be assistive and work under the direction of the registered nurse who remains accountable (SGNA, 2006). Preparation of the room and equipment is undertaken by the nurse in response to assessment of patient requirement and the procedure to be undertaken. Checks are conducted to ensure all relevant machinery is ready for use and in working order, so that the patient enters a calm and ordered environment. Equipment in the endoscopy room includes:

- Adjustable patient trolley
- Suction and oxygen equipment
- Pulse oximeter
- Resuscitation trolley
- Endoscopy trolley including the relevant endoscope, light source, camera and image apparatus, accessories, water/suction system
- Drugs and associated administration equipment
- Infection control protective devices such as gloves and aprons
  (Adapted from Radford, 2005, p. 246.)

As staff wear theatre attire introductions are made so that the patient is able to distinguish relevant personnel.

Patient preparation

Preliminary explanation of the procedure has been given through written communication and instructions for preparation. Patient preparation for lung and upper gastrointestinal procedures includes fasting for 8 hours pre-procedure and discontinuing anticoagulants, aspirin, proton pump inhibitors (PPIs) and non-steroidal anti-inflammatory drugs for 1 week prior to the procedure, or according to medical advice. For lower gastrointestinal examinations iron preparations also need to be stopped for at least a week and the bowel needs to be cleansed. This is achieved through following a liquid diet devoid of colourants and fat for 2 days. Items that may be consumed are:

- Clear soup
- Coffee and tea with skimmed milk
- Fruit juice that does not contain fruit pulp
- Gelatin
- Non-alcoholic drinks
- Water

On the day prior to the procedure a laxative preparation is taken, which causes diarrhoea and emptying of the bowel. Because of associated fluid loss it is important that patients continue to drink plenty of clear fluid to avoid dehydration.

Just prior to the procedure an intravenous cannula is inserted, usually by the nurse, so that intravenous medication can be given. Sedation and analgesia may be given in diagnostic examinations and are necessary for all therapeutic procedures. Where required, fluids may also be administered via this route. If more invasive techniques that breach the integrity of tissue are anticipated, or the patient is known to have a coagulopathy (clotting disorder), blood testing for clotting is also required prior to commencing procedures (Ogilvie et al., 2002). Patients are also assessed for the need for adjunct oxygen therapy during the procedure. For patients undergoing anal examinations a further consideration is the possibility of a history of having been abused. Giving permission for disclosure through ongoing communication and explanation and offering the opportunity for choice of care providers is one way to help patients to manage the procedure (Davy, 2006).

Aftercare

The priority of aftercare is observing for return of normal function and monitoring of vital signs as appropriate to the procedure, anaesthetic agent and drugs administered. Many patients will have fasted, or had a modified diet, beforehand and so are usually offered a snack with a drink if their swallowing is normal. When they are fully awake and recovered, an explanation of the findings of the examination is given and discussed with the patient by the nurse. Instruction is given for:

- Self-care
- Follow-up arrangements
- Any new medication prescribed
- Symptoms of complications to look out for
- When and where to seek further help

This provides an opportunity for further health education and health promotion. Patients are able to return home escorted by a responsible adult when fully recovered, or may return to their inpatient facility. If sedative, or anaesthetic, drugs have been administered patients should not operate machinery, make legal decisions, drink alcohol, take further sedatives, or drive for at least 24 hours. Onward referral to other members of the multidisciplinary team may be requested and needs to be facilitated by the nurse.

Care aspects of specific endoscopic procedures are as follows:

- Bronchoscopy – This procedure is used to visualise the bronchi of the lungs to obtain samples of secretions, or lung tissue, in the diagnosis of lung disease and cancer. The nasal or oral route may be used for insertion of the endoscope. Careful consideration needs to be given when using the nasal route if the patient has a deviated septum, or history of a broken nose, which could affect passing of the endoscope. Lignocaine lubricating gel is applied to the nostrils to aid the passage of the endoscope. When the oral route is used application of a bite block avoids damage occurring to the endoscope. Local anaesthetic spray, lignocaine, is administered to the back of the throat to anaesthetise the area regardless of the access route. Some patients are intubated under light anaesthetic if their condition, or the procedure, demands it. The examination usually takes up to an hour. Aftercare is determined by the drugs and level of anaesthetic administered. The priority of care is to maintain and monitor respiratory function through the use of a pulse oximeter and confirm the return of the gag reflex. Other vital signs such as pulse and blood pressure are also checked to ensure the adequacy of ventilation. Decision making revolves around identifying when patients are able to self-care and fit for discharge. It is important that patients do not eat or drink for 4–6 hours post-procedure and they need to be aware of this before becoming self-caring. Complications of bronchoscopy include bleeding due to tearing of the epithelial lining of the airways, or from biopsy sites, and aspiration pneumonia where material might be inhaled into the lower air passages on withdrawal of the endoscope. Patients may also have a hoarse voice for a while afterwards due to irritation of the vocal chords.

- Oesophagogastroduodenoscopy (OGD) – This procedure examines the oesophagus, stomach and duodenum to diagnose and treat disorders. It is indicated for pain on swallowing, determining the cause of gastrointestinal bleeding (particularly with unexplained anaemia), ulcer-type pain, dyspepsia accompanied by anorexia and weight loss, persistent nausea and vomiting and ulcer-type defects previously demonstrated with barium meal. Lignocaine spray is applied to the back of the throat and, depending on patient condition and choice, additional sedation may be administered intravenously. The patient is asked to accept the bite block and adopts the left lateral position with the head flexed forward to enable introduction of the endoscope (Ogilvie et al., 2002). Biopsies are taken of areas showing changes to ascertain reasons for the change.

  Therapeutic interventions include:
  - Dilatation of benign strictures such as scarring or for *achalasia* (reduced motility in the lower portion of the oesophagus and inability of the oesophageal or cardiac sphincter to relax and open and allow food to progress out of the oesophagus into the stomach)
  - Removal of foreign bodies or gastric polyps
  - Haemostasis of upper gastrointestinal bleeding caused by oesophageal varices or ulcers
  - *Stent* insertion (tube that keeps lumen walls open) and palliation of malignant tumours

  The diagnostic examination lasts about 20 min, but therapeutic ones may take considerably longer depending on anatomical structure and degree of disorder. Priorities of aftercare involve maintaining the patient on their side until fully recovered, including the return of the ability to swallow. Decision making relates to length of observation of vital signs, which is dependent on whether sedation has been administered, how patients recover from it and procedure complication risk. If there is increasing pain, or commencement of vomiting, the endoscopist is notified. Complications of the procedure include bleeding due to disruption of the lining of the stomach or duodenum and perforation of the actual wall.

Risks of perforation are greater when treating malignant lesions. Symptoms are exhibited as tachycardia and hypotension and a sharp increase in abdominal pain. The nurse reacts quickly in communicating and monitoring. Surgical opinion is usually sought and the patient admitted. Closed or confined perforation may be less obvious immediately but can become evident through the patient developing subcutaneous emphysema, which is air present in subcutaneous tissue. This is managed conservatively through keeping the patient nil by mouth, administering intravenous fluids and antibiotics (Cotton and Williams, 2003).

Opportunity for the student

Find out what the signs of subcutaneous (or surgical) emphysema are.

Infection may occur from contaminated equipment and haemostasis may cause necrosis of neighbouring tissue (American Society for Gastrointestinal Endoscopy (ASGE), 2002). It is important that patients are advised of warning signs of complications and when to seek further help from their general practitioner in order to self-manage while at home.

- Colonoscopy – This procedure examines the length of the large intestine starting from the anal canal and extending to the caecum and into the terminal ileum. It is indicated for investigating real or potential rectal bleeding, particularly in unexplained anaemia, changes in bowel habit, persistent unexplained abdominal pain, abnormalities found on barium enema such as a filling defect, follow-up after removal of bowel tumours and for some inflammatory bowel conditions. Diagnostic examination looks for signs of growths, such as polyps that arise from the lining of the bowel, for lesions such as *angiodysplasia* (capillary lesions in the colon walls that bleed) and for inflammation and ulceration. Colonoscopy is also useful to screen for colorectal cancer as part of a screening programme, although not all centres are currently in a position to offer this service due to high workload of the endoscopy service (Waye et al., 2004). The procedure itself takes up to an hour. Where cancers or cancerous polyps are found internal markers may be applied to aid follow-up surgical locating.

Therapeutic intervention is undertaken for:

- Excision of polyps
- Removal of foreign bodies
- Haemostasis through electrical coagulation
- Dilatation of stenosis
- Decompression of *volvulus* (where the bowel rotates causing obstruction)
- Palliation of tumours

The patient adopts the left lateral position because the descending and sigmoid colon are on the left, with knees drawn up towards the chest and bottom towards the edge of the couch as this aids insertion of the colonoscope (Ogilvie et al., 2002). Conscious sedation is administered with an opiate analgesic as this can be a painful procedure, but the patient may need to move during the examination to aid further advancement, particularly when nearing the caecum. Air is pumped into the bowel to separate the walls aiding visualisation. The colonoscope sometimes becomes looped, requiring the nurse to apply careful pressure to the abdomen to enable further advancement (Ogilvie et al., 2002).

Aftercare is directed at patient recovery from sedation, assessment of pain due to the air present in the bowel and monitoring for complications. Patients usually need to go to the toilet to expel air and should be accompanied as there is a risk of a vasovagal reaction causing temporary loss of consciousness (fainting). Complications associated with the procedure include bleeding and perforation. Perforation is more likely to occur in the small bowel where the wall is thinner. Bleeding may be delayed after polyp removal for up to 10 days. Secondary bleeding usually occurs after about 14 days and is evidenced by increasing frequency of bowel motions containing blood clots. Some patients may also develop 'polypectomy syndrome', which is exhibited by localised abdominal pain and mild fever due to the inflammatory response (Cotton and Williams, 2003).

- Sigmoidoscopy – This examines the lower portion of the large bowel including the anal canal, rectum, sigmoid colon and descending colon. It is indicated for investigating problems with elimination such as chronic diarrhoea or constipation, faecal incontinence and abnormal events such as rectal bleeding, rectal pain, ulceration as well as signs of abnormal growths and cancer. It is a more limited examination than colonoscopy, taking about 20 min. Aftercare and complications are similar to colonoscopy. Contraindications include active peritonitis, diverticulitis or recent bowel surgery (Cotton and Williams, 2003).

- Endoscopic retrograde cholangiopancreatogram (ERCP) – This procedure examines the bile and pancreatic ducts for disorders through a radiological image of the anatomy. It is usually undertaken in the radiology department because it involves both endoscopic and fluoroscopy visualisation, but can also carried out in an endoscopy unit with a lead-lined theatre. It may be diagnostic and therapeutic. It is indicated for removal of common bile duct stones, obstructive jaundice, undiagnosed upper abdominal pain, recurrent pancreatitis and cancer of the duct or pancreas (Ogilvie et al., 2003; Radford, 2005). Because radiopaque contrast is administered it is important to establish any allergies to iodine in advance, and the pregnancy status of female patients of reproductive age because of the radiation involved.

Cumulative knowledge

Why is an allergy to iodine of relevance? (Return to Chapter 7 on radiology nursing to check your answer.)

Antibiotics are always given prior to the procedure. The patient is positioned in the left lateral position to begin with. Conscious sedation, analgesia and often also an antispasmodic preparation to stop motility of the duodenal wall, are administered.

The endoscope is advanced through the oesophagus to the duodenum. A catheter filled with contrast dye is inserted into the papilla of the bile duct and dye is injected to outline the biliary and pancreatic ductal systems. X-rays are taken at this point and the patient rolled into the prone position to facilitate complete visualisation with further X-rays. If the duct is dilated, half-strength contrast is applied to avoid obscuring possible stones. If gallstones are located, it may be possible to remove them at this point. The duct is prepared for stone extraction using an electrocautery device called a *sphincterotome*, which makes an incision known as a *sphincterotomy* into the duct using electrical heat. A balloon-tipped catheter is used to draw the stones into the duodenum or a catheter with an expanding metal basket to trap and withdraw them completely. This then allows placement of a *stent* (a plastic tube that holds the duct walls open). Larger stones may require fragmenting through endoscopic pulsed laser to aid their retrieval. The procedure takes about an hour. Simple narrowing of the duct is dilated with dilators. Aftercare and complications are similar to OGD. Additional complication includes pancreatitis, which is evidenced by vomiting, pain and pyrexia.

- Percutaneous endoscopic gastrostomy (PEG) – In this procedure a feeding tube is inserted into the stomach through direct puncture under endoscopic visualisation and conscious sedation. It is indicated for disorders such as neurological dysphagia, malignancies of the head and neck and supplementary feeding for bowel conditions such as cystic fibrosis. Contraindications include oesophageal stricture, which precludes an endoscopic approach, requiring radiological placement instead. Prophylactic intravenous antibiotics are administered prior to the procedure.

The patient is placed in the supine position and the endoscope is passed into the stomach, which is then distended with air. The endoscope is aligned with the anterior wall of the stomach just above the umbilicus. Local anaesthetic is injected into the skin and external disinfectant preparation applied to the skin. The position is checked by external indentation confirmed by endoscopic viewing. An incision is made in the skin and a needle inserted to puncture the stomach wall. A snare passed through the accessories channel of the endoscope draws a wire, or suture thread, through the needle and up to the mouth. The PEG tube is connected to the wire/suture thread, drawn down and through the anterior stomach wall by an external loop of the wire/suture thread. The procedure takes about 20 min.

Complications include peritonitis, wound infection, seeding of malignancies and tube dislodgement. Those with neurological problems will require close observation of the airway to avoid aspiration problems during the procedure. It is important to keep PEG tubes patent through flushing with water before and after insertion of other liquids.

- Transoesophageal echocardiogram (TOE) – This procedure is undertaken to examine the chambers, valves and blood vessels of the heart. Indications for the examination include diagnosing disorders of the heart valves, hole in the heart, endocarditis and thrombosis. The endoscope is tipped with an ultrasound probe and advanced to the part of the oesophagus which lies behind the heart. Ultrasound images of blood flowing through the heart and its beating function are conveyed to a monitor and reviewed by a specialist.

Contrast may be administered intravenously to add clarity to the images of blood flow. This contains microbubbles of gas which alter reflection of the sonic wave (Deklunder, 2002). Because the bubble wall is composed of albumin, allergy to egg is a precluding factor to its use and needs to be ascertained beforehand. The procedure takes about 15 min. Aftercare is similar to OGD in terms of recovering normal function and consciousness where sedation has been given. Complications include perforation of the oesophagus and bleeding.

Opportunity for the student

Find out about any additional procedures not listed here that might be available in your placement area. What is the nursing role?

Developing role

The nurse sedationist

Sedation is given for many endoscopic procedures. Levels are determined by the likelihood of discomfort, patient history, patient anxiety and procedural requirement for immobility or ventilatory respiratory support. Sedation can be categorised as:

- Minimal – drug-induced relaxed condition to combat anxiety
- Moderate – the patient being able to consciously respond to commands accompanied by tactile rousing
- Deep sedation – consciousness depressed, requiring sustained tactile rousing and some respiratory support
- General anaesthetic – drug-induced loss of consciousness requiring ventilatory support (SGNA, 2004a)

Nurses who have undertaken specialised training and preparation in assessment, pharmacology, patient monitoring, airway management and advanced life support are now able to undertake the sedationist role to support deep-level sedation (SGNA, 2004b). For minimal and moderate levels of sedation they can administer drugs prescribed by a doctor and for deep level of sedation they administer drugs under the supervision of a doctor (SGNA, 2004a). General anaesthetics are only administered by anaesthetists. Sedation is titrated according to patient response, the desired level of sedation and risks posed by effects of the drug. The nurse continually monitors these effects by observing the patient and monitoring vital signs throughout the procedure and into the recovery phase. It is recommended that the nurse monitors patient sedation and its effects during procedures in lieu of other activity (SGNA, 2004a).

Opportunity for the student

What drugs are used for sedation in your placement area?
What are their pharmacological effects and reversal agents?

The nurse endoscopist

The modernisation agenda (Department of Health – CNO's Directorate, 2006) expects nurses to develop new competencies and transfer skills to work across occupational boundaries. Patient, rather than profession need, is at the centre of who provides care. The nurse endoscopist is one such role development of advancing practice meeting the rising demand for endoscopy services. In order to complete additional preparation and training, nurses need to have a length of experience of working in an endoscopy unit, be able to undertake study at level 3, have a good knowledge of anatomy, physiology, pathophysiology, pharmacology and have a good understanding of medicolegal issues. Specialist courses are offered by certified centres and underwritten by associated education partner institutions (Pathmakanthan et al., 2001). A period of supervised practice is undertaken within recognised placements with competency assessed by a practising endoscopist. Nurses have been found to be as competent as their medical colleagues in carrying out procedures (British Society of Gastroenterology Decontamination Working Group, 2005b).

The range of examinations that nurses undertake has gradually expanded from diagnostic to include the therapeutic, such as oesophageal dilatation, polypectomy, stent and PEG insertions. But, ERCP remains within the medical domain and only a few centres venture into variceal injection. Prescribing of medication is under a patient group direction which is a written direction signed by a doctor and by a pharmacist relating to administration of specified medications to a defined group of people who meet certain criteria. These developments and blurring of boundaries have led to regulatory bodies starting to reassess what is meant by advanced practice (Nursing and Midwifery Council (NMC), 2007).

Future developments

It is likely that nurses will continue to take on the full range of services offered by the medical endoscopist as their experience and practice expand. Consultant nurses already exist in other fields of practice, such as intensive care and renal services, and it seems likely that the nurse endoscopist may be able to use transferable skills to translate practice to a higher level of autonomy. The modernisation agenda (DH, 2006) requires services to be located closer to the patient and this may provide nurses an opportunity to become even more independent.

Scenario

Mrs Chacko is 54 years old and a Hindu. She speaks no English. She presented to outpatients with a history of tiredness and unexplained anaemia and was referred, by the consultant, for a gastroscopy. She is accompanied by her husband who speaks good English.

(1) What are the priorities for this woman's care?
(2) How do you manage her confidentiality?

Summary

As technology has developed a greater variety of patients and conditions have presented for diagnostic and therapeutic intervention. Endoscopy nursing has followed developments in this field of practice, with nurses increasingly taking on roles previously undertaken by other professionals. Opportunities for the student have been highlighted in developing knowledge of decontamination techniques, types of sedatives and their reversal agents and the scope of procedures and practice. Reflection on physiological knowledge enables students to respond critically to emergent situations in the aftercare of patients.

Acknowledgement

Although the author is responsible for the text, she acknowledges the contribution of Ian Coates, previously Endoscopy Charge Nurse QEQMH and currently Outpatient Manager, Spencer Wing, for checking the accuracy of the text and proof reading the work.

Glossary of terms

Achalasia
Condition of reduced motility emptying of the oesophagus

Angiodysplasia
Capillary lesions in the bowel wall that bleed

Coagulopathy
Clotting disorder

Endoscopy
Visualisation of the inside of body tracts

Proton pump inhibitor
Reduces the production of hydrochloric acid

Sphincterotome
Electrocautery device for cutting using electrical heat

Sphincterotomy
Incision in a sphincter or duct

Surgical emphysema
Air present within subcutaneous tissue

Stent
Metal mesh or plastic tube structure to hold lumen walls apart

Vasovagal
Response of the involuntary vagus nerve that slows the heart rate causing hypotension often stimulated in relation to straining against a closed glottis

Volvulus
Rotation of the bowel blocking off the lumen

Websites

http://www.asge.org
http://www.bsg.org.uk
http://www.18weeks.nhs.uk/public/default.aspx?main=true&load=ArticleViewer
&ArticleId=565
http://www.sgna.org/

References

American Society for Gastrointestinal Endoscopy (2002) Complications of upper GI endoscopy. *Gastrointestinal Endoscopy* 55(7), pp. 784–793.

Association of Perioperative Registered Nurses (2003) Recommended Practices for cleaning and processing endoscopes and endoscopic accessories. *AORN Journal* 77(2), pp. 434–438, 441–442.

Breier-Mackie, S. (2005) Ethics and endoscopy. *Gastroenterology Nursing* 28(6), pp. 514–515.

British Society of Gastroenterology Decontamination Working Group (2005a) *Endoscopy and Individuals at Risk of vCJD for Public Health Purposes.* London: British Society of Gastroenterology.

British Society of Gastroenterology Decontamination Working Group (2005b) *Non-Medical Endoscopists* [online]. Available from: http://ww.bsg.org.uk/pdf_word_docs/endo_%20nonmed.pdf (accessed 29 June 2007).

British Society of Gastroenterology Working Party Report (2003, updated 2005) *Guidelines for Decontamination of Equipment for Gastrointestinal Endoscopy.* London: British Society of Gastroenterology.

Cotton, P.B. and Williams, C.B. (2003) *Practical Gastrointestinal Endoscopy: The Fundamentals,* 5th ed. Oxford: Blackwell Publishing.

Davy, E. (2006) The endoscopy patient with a history of sexual abuse: strategies for compassionate care. *Gastroenterology Nursing* 29(3), pp. 221–225.

Deklunder, G. (2002) Role of ultrasound and contrast enhanced ultrasound in patients with cerebrovascular disease. *European Heart Journal Supplements* 4(Suppl. C), pp. C51–C55.

Glenn, T. (2001) Esophageal cancer: facts, figures and screening. *Gastroenterology Nursing* 24(6), 271–273.

Department of Health (2000a) *The NHS Plan.* London: HMSO.

Department of Health (2000b) *The NHS Cancer Plan A Plan for Investment A Plan for Reform.* London: HMSO.

Department of Health (2003) *Guide to the Decontamination of Reusable Surgical Instruments.* London: HMSO.

Department of Health (2004) *The NHS Improvement Plan.* London: HMSO.

Department of Health – CNO's Directorate (2006) *Modernising Nursing Careers: Setting the Direction.* London: HMSO.

Jacobson, D. and Katzman, P. (2001) *Benefits of Xenon Technology for Machine Vision Illumination* [online]. Santa Clara, CA: PerkinElmer Optoelectronics Inc. Available from: http://optoelectronics.perkinelmer.com/content/RelatedLinks/Articles/ATL_myarticles.pdf (accessed 12 June 2007).

Macari, M. and Bini, E.J. (2005) CT colonography: where have we been and where are we going? *Radiology 237*, pp. 819–833.

Medicines and Healthcare products Regulatory Agency (MHRA) (2006) *Top Ten Tips Endoscope Decontamination*. London: Medicines and Healthcare products Regulatory Agency.

National Audit Office (2005) *Department of Health: The NHS Cancer Plan: A Progress Report*. London: The Audit Office.

National Institute for Health and Clinical Excellence (NIHCE) (2006) *Patient Safety and the Reduction of Risk of Transmission of Creutzfelt-Jakob(CJD) Disease via Interventional Procedures*. London: National Institute for Clinical Excellence.

Nursing and Midwifery Council (NMC) (2007) *Advanced Nursing Practice – Update19 June 2007* [online]. Available from: http://www.nmc-uk.org/aArticle.aspx?ArticleID=2528 (accessed 20 June 2007).

Ogilvie, J., Norwitz, L. and Kalloo, A. (2002) *The John Hopkins Manual for Intestinal Endoscopy Nursing*. New Jersey: Slack Incorporated.

Pathmakanthan, S., Murray, I., Smith, K., Heeley, R. and Donnelly, M. (2001) Nurse endoscopists in United Kingdom health care: a survey of prevalence, skills and attitudes. *Journal of Advanced Nursing 36*(5), pp. 705–710.

Radford, M. (2005) Surgery outside the operating department, in Woodhead, K. and Wicker, P. (eds) *A Textbook of Perioperative Care*. Edinburgh: Elsevier Churchill Livingstone, pp. 229–250.

Social Care Institute for Excellence (2007) *Practice Guide 09. Dignity in Care* [online]. Available from: http://www.scie.org.uk/publications/practiceguides/practiceguide09/index.asp (accessed 2 October 2007).

Society of Gastroenterology Nurses and Associates Inc (SGNA) (2003) *Guidelines for Documentation in the Gastrointestinal Endoscopy Setting* [online]. Available from: http://www.sgna.org/Resources/guidelines/guideline7.cfm (accessed 20 June 2007).

Society of Gastroenterology Nurses and Associates Inc (2004a) Position statement: statement on the use of sedation and analgesia in the gastrointestinal endoscopy setting. *Gastroenterology Nursing 27*(3), pp. 142–144.

Society of Gastroenterology Nurses and Associates Inc (2004b) Position statement: ASGE/SGNA Role of GI registered nurses in the management of patients undergoing sedation procedures [online]. Available from: http://www.sgna.org/Resources/statements/jointstatement.cfm (accessed 29 June 2007).

Society of Gastroenterology Nurses and Associates Inc (2005) *Standards of Clinical Nursing Practice and Role Delineation Statements* [online]. Available from: http://www.sgna.org/Resources/guidelines/guideline8.cfm (accessed 20 June 2007).

Society of Gastroenterology Nurses and Associates Inc (2006) Position statement: Minimal registered nurse staffing [online]. Available from: http://www.sgna.org/resources/statements/statement14.cfm (accessed 20 June 2007).

Waye, J.D., Rex, D.K. and Williams, C.B. (2004) *Colonoscopy – Principles and Practice*. Oxford: Blackwell Publishing.

Chapter 9

Perioperative care in day surgery

Beverley McNeil

Learning objectives
After reading this chapter and participating in the activities, the reader should have a clearer understanding of:

- Preparation of the patient for theatre
- The importance of gaining informed consent
- Different types of anaesthetics and methods of induction
- The roles and responsibilities of theatre practitioners
- The function of the recovery room
- The process of discharge from the day surgery unit

Introduction

Definition of day surgery

Patients are carefully pre-assessed for suitability for day surgery, otherwise known as 'ambulatory surgery', and then admitted to hospital for a scheduled surgical procedure, which may or may not require general anaesthesia, and full operating theatre facilities (though both are available). Providing discharge criteria are met, the patient will return home within 24 hours with pre-arranged support.

In recent years a significant increase in day surgery provision has been witnessed within the United Kingdom (UK), with some trusts increasing day case rates by 6–10% within a single year. Monetary and political drivers for change place the focus of attention firmly on ambulatory surgery, whilst the creation of 33 new National Health Service (NHS) treatment centres and 22 independent-sector treatment centres have helped increase overall capacity within the service (Department of Health (DH), 2007a; McMillan, 2005).

Patient satisfaction with day surgery combined with significant advances in anaesthesia and surgery continues to propel expansion (DH, 2005). Shorter acting drugs for general anaesthesia, the use of local and regional anaesthetic techniques and improved management of pain and postoperative nausea and vomiting (PONV) all contribute to the patient experiencing minimal side effects and a more rapid recovery from surgery. Surgery itself has been revolutionised by advances in instrumentation, such as laparoscopic equipment, flexible endoscopes, lasers and harmonic scalpels. Other developments have decreased operating time, e.g. the diathermy hand-switching pencil, which allows body tissues to be dissected quickly with minimal blood loss, and skin clips, which hasten skin closure for many surgical procedures.

Developments in medical devices and surgical technique therefore make it possible for increasingly complex procedures to be undertaken within the day surgery milieu, resulting in a continual challenging of traditional ways of working. The Association for Perioperative Practice (AfPP) (formerly the National Association of Theatre Nurses (NATN)) suggests that exactly the same facilities are necessary for day surgery as are provided within a main theatre suite, and day surgery should not be thought of 'as a subspecialty of surgery' (Beesley and Pirie, 2004, p. 219).

Utilisation of main theatre complexes and inpatient wards for day surgery tends to be associated with last-minute cancellations as acute and trauma patients take precedence over elective cases. Therefore day surgery is best provided within purpose-built units, thus ensuring the proximity of amenities and prevention of last-minute cancellations (Beesley and Pirie, 2004; British Association of Day Surgery (BADS), 2003).

The government target that no one need wait more than 18 weeks for treatment following referral by a general practitioner (GP) will further intensify the need for day surgery. In revising the basket of procedures suitable for undertaking on a day case basis, the Audit Commission suggests that 75% of 25 specified surgical procedures should be possible as day cases. This would free up 39 000 bed days, and based on a cost of £200 per elective bed day, would result in savings of £78 million. Currently in excess of 90% of cataract extractions are undertaken on a day case basis. From 2008, patients will be able to select whether to have their operation performed within NHS Acute Trusts, Foundation Trusts, independent-sector treatment centres or approved independent-sector hospitals (DH, 2007a). Given greater choice and acknowledging patient preference for day surgery, demand for the service is only likely to increase.

Day surgery requires experienced practitioners who are energised by the fast pace of the work and challenged by the variety of procedures undertaken. Expert communication skills are also necessary in order that a therapeutic relationship can be established with the patient in a short space of time (Rogan Foy and Timmins, 2004). The day surgery unit will be staffed with operating department practitioners (ODPs), nurses and health care assistants. Whilst multi-skilled staff are an advantage within a day surgery unit, ODPs and nurses often gravitate to one specialist area, either anaesthetics, theatre (scrub/circulating role) or recovery. The aim of this chapter is to give the reader a broad overview of the work undertaken by the multidisciplinary team within a day surgery unit, through documenting the care requirements of patients systematically progressing through their perioperative journey.

Admission and preparation of the patient for surgery

Staggered admission times are advocated with a view to reducing the patient's wait for surgery (McMillan, 2005). This also reduces temporary congestion and creates an impression of a well-organised unit. On arrival the patient should be greeted in a calm, professional manner, thus helping to instil confidence and alleviate natural apprehension regarding the forthcoming procedure. Many patients attending for day surgery will feel that matters are beyond their control. Patient empowerment is therefore essential. This can be achieved by ascertaining and then enhancing what the patient already knows, identifying needs and allowing participation in decision making, whilst making it clear that within a day surgery unit, the patient will take a degree of responsibility for his/her own care (Rogan Foy and Timmins, 2004). Hence, good communication skills, the ability to interpret body language and establishment of rapport are fundamental in helping allay patient fears and in eliciting last-minute information.

> **Cumulative knowledge**
>
> Both verbal and non-verbal methods of effective communication with anxious patients can be found within Chapter 2.

Generally, a named nurse/ODP will admit the patient, obtaining baseline readings of pulse and blood pressure for documentation within the local integrated care pathway (ICP) document commenced at pre-assessment (BADS, 2004a) (see the section on ICPs in Chapter 6 – Preoperative assessment in day surgery). Patients are advised of an appropriate fasting regime at pre-assessment, and it is the responsibility of the admitting practitioner to document the time the patient last ate and drank. Surgery may involve administration of a sedative or general anaesthetic at which time the patient's ability to communicate is compromised. In the event the patient is unable to provide his/her own details, the multidisciplinary team will need to rely solely on patient information contained within the ICP during the perioperative period. Careful documentation including comorbidities, allergies and prostheses is therefore essential.

Fasting

Preoperative fasting is undertaken to minimise the risk of aspiration of gastric contents during the perioperative period. Frequently, and for a variety of reasons, last-minute changes are made to the order of the operating list. To accommodate last-minute alterations and ensure all patients are potentially ready to be first on the operating list, a situation has arisen whereby 'convenience' or ritualistic fasting is commonplace. This results in patients fasting for much longer than is necessary, with many patients scheduled for surgery on a morning list consuming their last meal the evening prior to surgery. International guidelines (American Society of Anesthesiologists, 1999), however, promote the adequacy of fasting adult patients who are about to undergo general anaesthesia, regional anaesthesia or sedation/analgesia for:

- 8 hours – Fried/fatty foods/meat
- 6 hours – Light carbohydrate meal (toast/biscuits/tea)
- 2 hours – Clear fluid (water/fruit juice without pulp/tea or coffee without milk)

And infants for:

- 6 hours – food/non-human milk
- 4 hours – breast milk
- 2 hours – clear fluid

Ideally then, patient fasting should be individualised and where surgery is scheduled for the afternoon list it is marginally easier to stagger fast times appropriately. Advice to consume a light carbohydrate breakfast is given since fat, protein and meat take longer to digest.

Opportunity for the student

As the scope of day surgery extends to cover many specialities and a wider range of procedures, an increase is noted in the numbers of children and young people admitted. A comprehensive day surgery information sheet compiled by the Royal College of Nursing (2004) details comprehensive guidance on the care needs of this client group (http://www.rcn.org.uk/publications/pdf/daysurgery_cyp.pdf).

Access this information and answer the following critical review questions:

- Why are prolonged starvation periods avoided in children?
- Is it still acceptable for children to receive intramuscular injections?

Preoperative shaving

Controversy regarding preoperative shaving continues. The World Health Organization (2006) recommends shaving patients immediately prior to surgery since this is associated with reduced surgical site infection (SSI) rates (3.1%), when compared with shaving the day before surgery (7.1%). Microscopic breaks in the skin surface permit microbial colonisation of the proposed incision area, allowing SSI rates to rise to 20% where shaving occurs more than 24 hours in advance of surgery (Pyrek, 2007). However, a recent Cochrane Collaboration review on preoperative shaving (Tanner et al., 2006) concluded that there was no evidence to suggest that SSIs increased as a result of shaving the day before surgery. All studies were in agreement that if body hair must be removed prior to surgery, then depilatory agents and electric clippers resulted in less SSIs than razors.

Allergies/prostheses

Allergies will be confirmed by the admitting practitioner, since this may influence the anaesthetic administered, medication and, in some circumstances, the fluids and equipment utilised intra-operatively. Currently the patient may be given an allergy band as opposed to or in addition to a routine name band. Standardisation of information, design and the process of checking wristbands will reduce the potential for adverse incidents and thereby enhance patient safety. Thus following recommendations from the National Patient Safety Agency (NPSA) standardisation of wristbands will commence in July of 2008 (National Patient Safety Agency (NPSA), 2007; StaffNurse.com, 2007). Latex allergies should be communicated to theatre as early in proceedings as possible, to allow the multidisciplinary team to substitute latex-free anaesthetic and intra-operative equipment in advance of the patient's arrival. Equally important, metal prostheses (e.g. hip implants and screws/plates), deformities and stiffness of limbs (such as osteoarthritis) must be documented, since additional precautions may be necessary in the transfer and positioning of patients on the operating table.

Informed consent

Generally, consent to perform the proposed surgery will be obtained by the operating surgeon, just prior to commencing the morning or afternoon list. He/she will visit the day surgery ward and gain consent from each patient individually. It is the responsibility of the named nurse/ODP to ensure this happens. In some circumstances, consent will have been obtained during the initial outpatient consultation. Since consent is an ongoing process, where a significant amount of time has elapsed since this was first obtained, it will be necessary to ascertain that the patient is still consenting to treatment (General Medical Council, 2006).

Historically, informed consent (the patient's authorisation of an intervention) has been problematical; complicated as it is with both legal and ethical considerations (Beauchamp and Childress, 1994). Four types of consent forms are available for differing circumstances, ranging from consent for minors, through to adults who are unable to consent for themselves (DH, 2007b). Theatre practitioners should therefore be conversant with the form to use in differing circumstances. Those working within a day surgery unit should appreciate that consent must be gained in advance of the administration of any anaesthetic drugs and prior to the administration of any treatment to the patient. Pre-medication of the patient occurs rarely in day surgery because of its residual sedative effects. However, when a 'pre-med' is used, consent must be gained before and not after its administration.

Opportunity for the student

Check out the DH (2007b) website. Available from http://www.dh.gov.uk/en/Policyandguid-ance/ Healthandsocialcaretopics/Consent/Consentgeneralinformation/index.htm.
   Familiarise yourself with the guidance given to patients prior to signing their consent form and identify differences in the four consent forms available.

Traditionally, when gaining consent it was sufficient for a doctor to give the patient an account of the forthcoming procedure. More recently, the focus has shifted somewhat, so that in addition to disclosing information the quality of the patient's understanding of the explanation is paramount. Beauchamp and Childress (2001, p. 80) identify seven important elements which are necessary before consent can be termed 'informed'. (*Words in italics are supplied by the author.*)

(1) Competence (*the wherewithal to understand the procedure and decide upon it*)
(2) Voluntariness (*that the decision may be made without duress*)
(3) Disclosure (*a comprehensive explanation of the material information regarding the procedure has been given by the surgeon including the benefits, risks and alternatives*)
(4) Recommendation (*a plan of care has been outlined*)
(5) Understanding (*the patient has understood both the explanation of the procedure and the proposed plan*)
(6) Decision (*the patient chooses in favour of the plan*)
(7) Authorisation (*the patient sanctions the plan which has been outlined and agrees to proceed with treatment*)

Consent is best obtained by the individual undertaking the procedure in order that a thorough explanation can be given and questions may be answered. However, it is acceptable for a colleague to substitute, provided they too are capable of performing the operation. In certain circumstances other members of the health care team are specially trained to seek consent for specific procedures. Patients may withdraw consent at any time during the perioperative journey and this decision must be respected by all staff (NHS Modernisation Agency, 2002).

An explanation should be given regarding what the procedure involves – the benefits and the likelihood of obtaining them. Alternatives to the procedure should be conveyed along with the risks involved – whether these are serious or minor and what will happen should the procedure not proceed (NHS Modernisation Agency, 2002).

The anaesthetist will also visit the patient just prior to surgery when the type of anaesthesia to be administered will be discussed. The patient is supplied with a hospital gown and then jewellery (apart from a wedding ring which is taped to prevent inadvertent loss), dentures and contact lenses are removed. Where glasses and/or a hearing aid are worn, these may accompany the patient to theatre to aid with communication and help maintain patient dignity. Patients are encouraged to walk to theatre, though wheelchairs and trolleys are also utilised (McEwen, 2003). Innovations in the latter have resulted in day surgery trolleys which double as operating tables bringing significant benefits in reduced moving and handling as well as transfer time.

Induction of anaesthesia

On arrival at the theatre reception/holding area, and prior to transfer to the anaesthetic room, the patient will once again be taken through the preoperative checklist and consent form to ensure preparation for surgery is complete. Patients undergoing a surgical or invasive procedure will require either general, regional or local anaesthesia, or conscious sedation. A member of the perioperative team, either an ODP or a nurse with a post-registration anaesthetic qualification, will assist the anaesthetist within the anaesthetic room.

It is perhaps useful at this point to clarify the terms analgesia and anaesthesia. Both are derived from the Greek language, with *analgesia* meaning 'without pain' and '*anaesthesia*' indicating 'without feeling/sensation'. Within a day surgery unit, the aim is to tailor the type of anaesthesia used to the needs of the patient and the type of procedure. For example nerve blocks are increasingly used within day surgery to prevent transmission of pain impulses from limbs and certain areas of the body, thus doing away with the need for general anaesthesia and facilitating a faster recovery. In these circumstances it is common to hear the terms 'regional anaesthesia' or 'regional analgesia' being used interchangeably (Simpson and Popat, 2002).

General anaesthesia

Pharmacological agents are employed to induce the 'triad' of anaesthesia which comprises *narcosis* (hypnosis or sleep), analgesia (pain relief) and relaxation (paralysis of muscles). Narcosis, analgesia and relaxation are basic requirements for successful *balanced anaesthesia*, though proportions of each element will differ in relation to the procedure to be undertaken (Simpson and Popat, 2002). Thus deep, moderate or light anaesthesia can be achieved. General anaesthesia can be induced intravenously whereby a rapid bolus dose of the anaesthetic agent is administered and takes effect within one arm–brain circulation time. One arm–brain circulation time is the time taken for the anaesthetic drug injected into a vein in the back of the hand, or arm, to pass through the circulatory system and begin to have its effect upon the brain (usually 20–30 sec). Propofol has become one of the most popular intravenous induction agents in day surgery since it results in rapid unconsciousness, recovery within 4–6 min with no 'hangover' effects (Whelan and Davies, 2000).

Inhalational anaesthetic agents are slightly slower to take effect but are equally effective in inducing anaesthesia. They are less frequently used in adults nowadays as a result of anaesthesia provider and patient preference for rapid intravenous induction (Phillips, 2004). However, inhalational induction is still commonly utilised for young children, particularly those averse to the discomfort of intravenous cannula insertion preoperatively and for those with needle phobias (De-Lamar, 2003). Inhalational agents are volatile halogenated hydrocarbons such as halothane, enflurane, isoflurane, sevoflurane and desflurane which are administered through a vaporiser. At induction, the volatile agent in combination with nitrous oxide (the only true gas used for anaesthesia) is inhaled, along with oxygen, via a face mask (Phillips, 2004). The molecules of the volatile agent diffuse across capillary membranes of the alveoli, enter the bloodstream and are subsequently transported to the brain where they have their anaesthetic effect (Griffiths, 2000).

The action by which either intravenous or inhalational anaesthetic agents induce anaesthesia is not completely understood. It is recognised, however, that the central nervous system is the main site of action and when an adequate amount of the anaesthetic agent reaches the cerebral cortex and binds with neurone cell membranes, the ability of these nerve cells to convey electrical activity is inhibited and thus association pathways are broken. The result is virtually complete cessation of sensory perception, motor discharge and an 'unconscious' patient who is quiet, immobile and who will have no recollection of surgery (Phillips, 2004).

Once induction of general anaesthesia has occurred, unconsciousness results and the patient's ability to maintain a patent airway and breathe normally become compromised. This necessitates insertion of a breathing tube through which the intraoperative administration of selected anaesthetic agents occurs. A certain amount of relaxation is generally necessary prior to insertion of the breathing tube and relaxation is induced by administration of an intravenous injection of a muscle relaxant.

Muscle relaxants prevent transmission of impulses from motor nerves to skeletal muscles, thus producing a temporary paralysis or relaxation of muscles. Invariably, a short-acting muscle relaxant will be used at commencement of the induction process to facilitate insertion of the breathing tube. During some forms of surgery (particularly when the surgeon needs access to tight body cavities), a long-acting muscle relaxant can be administered at regular intervals intra-operatively. This will produce prolonged muscle relaxation and thus optimum working conditions. With the exclusion of the heart, muscle relaxants affect all muscles of the body, including the accessory muscles of respiration and the diaphragm; thus, it becomes necessary to mechanically ventilate the patient. At this time, while the patient is unable to breathe for him/herself, this normal bodily function is taken over by a mechanical ventilator under the close supervision of anaesthetic staff; hence, care is termed 'wholly compensatory' (Phillips, 2004).

For a paralysed patient, the breathing tube of choice is an endotracheal (ET) tube (see Figure 9.1), although the laryngeal mask airway (LMA) is now considered an acceptable alternative in certain circumstances. Using an illuminated blade laryngoscope, the ET tube is inserted into the oropharynx and under direct vision guided between the vocal cords into the trachea. An ET tube may be composed of silicone, plastic or metal and has an integral cuff which is inflated following satisfactory positioning. The cuff prevents inadvertent aspiration of gastric contents should gastroesophageal reflux occur, thus protecting the lungs from contamination with surgical debris. Once taped or tied into position externally, the tube provides a

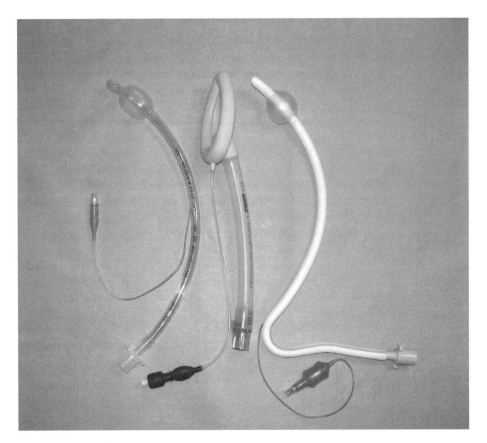

Figure 9.1 Anaesthetic breathing tubes. From right to left: endotracheal tube, laryngeal mask and nasal tube. [Photograph – Beverley McNeil.]

secure airway for the delivery of intra-operative gases. For intra-oral surgery it will be necessary to utilise a nasal tube (see Figure 9.1) (Ince et al., 2000).

An alternative to the ET tube is the LMA (see Figure 9.1) – a flexible tube with an oval inflatable cuff designed to sit over the larynx. Introduced via the mouth and correctly positioned and inflated, the space around and behind the larynx is completely occluded, forming a continuation between tube and trachea. Protective effects against aspiration and regurgitation are considerably reduced; hence, this form of airway is not suitable for all patients and surgical positions; however, ease and speed of insertion for low-risk patients undergoing day surgery procedures have made LMAs the most popular method of securing the airway within day surgery units (Phillips, 2004).

Whichever method of induction and type of breathing tube is employed, maintenance of anaesthesia will normally consist of the intra-operative administration of oxygen, with either air or nitrous oxide and a volatile agent (Simpson and Popat, 2002). However, total intravenous anaesthesia using an infusion of propofol is possible where adverse reactions to volatile agents might be a possibility, e.g. in the case of malignant hyperthermia (McNeil, 2005).

Once anaesthesia has been induced and the airway secured, the patient will be transferred from the anaesthetic room into the operating theatre for commencement of the procedure. Unless surgery is to be undertaken on the existing trolley, transfer onto the operating table will occur. Careful intra-operative monitoring of the patient throughout the procedure is essential; therefore, electrocardiographic (ECG) monitoring is attached along with a blood pressure cuff and pulse oximetry probe.

Regional anaesthesia

General anaesthesia is not without its risks, especially for patients with comorbidities such as cardiovascular disease. Frequently, surgery within a day surgery unit is performed under regional rather than general anaesthesia, with the benefit that the patient may remain awake, conscious and cooperative throughout the procedure. The purpose of regional anaesthesia is thus to bring about a loss of sensation in a particular area of the body in order to facilitate surgery without inducing unconsciousness. This involves infiltration of a local anaesthetic agent (e.g. a levobupivacaine such as Chirocaine) around a particular nerve or group of nerves distant from the surgical site, but comprising the sensory pathways supplying the area. Pain impulses from the surgical site are therefore interrupted or blocked. Regional 'blocks' are utilised for fairly extensive procedures, and nerve blocks, spinal anaesthesia, epidural anaesthesia and Bier's blocks all fall into the category of regional anaesthesia.

Nerve blocks

A local anaesthetic solution (e.g. Xylocaine or Chirocaine) is injected close to the nerve or nerves supplying the intended site of operation, thus blocking nerve supply to the area and therefore pain sensation (e.g. the brachial plexus supplying the arm) (Potter and Perry, 2005).

Spinal anaesthesia

Spinal anaesthesia (or intrathecal block) involves a lumbar puncture and a single injection of a small volume (2–3 mL) of the anaesthetic agent (often heavy bupivacaine) into cerebrospinal fluid (CSF) contained within the spinal subarachnoid space. The subarachnoid space lies between the pia mater and arachnoid mater, which constitute the inner two layers of the meninges surrounding the spinal cord (see Figure 9.2). Desensitisation or 'numbing' of spinal ganglia and motor nerve roots occurs and because the position of the patient will influence distribution of the liquid anaesthetic agent, these patients should not be unintentionally 'tilted' or inadvertent paralysis of respiratory muscles may occur (Phillips, 2004).

Spinal anaesthesia, commonly referred to as a 'spinal', is used relatively infrequently in day surgery but is extremely useful for lower extremity procedures and

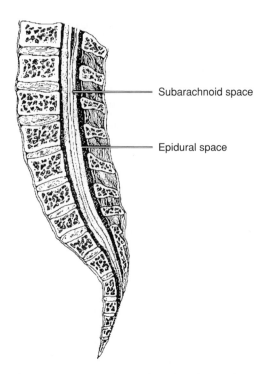

Subarachnoid space

Epidural space

Figure 9.2 Local anaesthetic agent is injected into subarachnoid space for spinal anaesthesia or into epidural space for epidural anaesthesia. [Reproduced from *Berry and Kohn's Operating Room Technique*, 10th ed. Phillips, 2004, p. 430, with permission from Elsevier.]

for abdominal, pelvic and urological operations (Potter and Perry, 2005). Spinal anaesthesia will be effective for approximately 4 hours, so care must be taken to ensure complete regression of the block and full return of motor and sensory function before the patient is discharged from the day surgery unit (BADS, 2004b).

Epidural anaesthesia

Epidural anaesthesia also involves injecting between the lumber vertebrae but this time with a larger volume of the anaesthetic agent (10–20 mL of bupivacaine), into the epidural space lying between dura mater, the outer layer of the meninges and the ligaments supporting the vertebral column (see Figure 9.2). This is a marginally safer procedure than spinal anaesthesia because the anaesthetic agent does not puncture CSF but targets the space outside the dura mater. Therefore, while the depth of anaesthesia can be just as profound as with spinal anaesthesia, onset will take longer as the anaesthetic agent slowly diffuses through the epidural space and penetrates the nerve roots as they leave the spinal cord. Unlike spinals, anaesthetic distribution will not be influenced by the patient's position (Phillips, 2004).

Whilst spinals involve a 'one-off' injection of a local anaesthetic solution, epidurals allow the option of inserting a catheter into the epidural space for 'top-ups' to

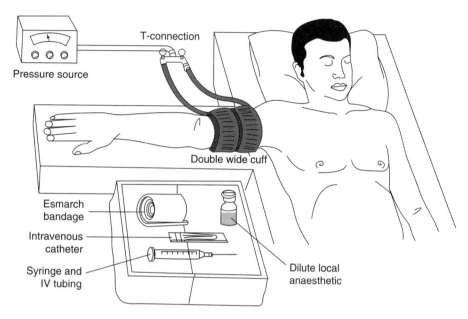

Figure 9.3 Biers block. [Reprinted from *Berry and Kohn's Operating Room Technique*, 10th edn. Phillips, 2004, with permission from Elsevier.]

be given. Since epidural catheters may remain in position for up to 5 days, analgesic effects can be prolonged well into the postoperative period, which is useful following major surgery. In day surgery, however, they are removed following the procedure. Epidural anaesthesia is frequently used for vaginal, perineal and obstetric procedures (Potter and Perry, 2005).

Bier's block (intravenous regional anaesthesia)

A double-cuffed (proximal and distal cuff) tourniquet is applied to an extremity and intravenous access is gained (see Figure 9.3). The limb is exsanguinated. (Blood is removed by elevation of the limb or application of an Esmarch (rubber) bandage or device to compress the limb with the aim of squeezing blood back towards the trunk or 'core' of the body.) The proximal cuff (nearest the core) is inflated. The local anaesthetic agent (often prilocaine) is injected via the intravenous cannula and once analgesia is achieved within the limb, the distal cuff (most distant from the core) is inflated, and the proximal cuff then deflated. The tourniquet is now positioned on a 'numbed' portion of the limb, thus reducing discomfort from the inflated cuff. Tourniquets must be released after an absolute maximum of 2 hours to prevent damage to the limb. Cells within a limb deprived of circulating oxygen will have metabolised anaerobically, producing lactic acid. Once the tourniquet is released, the patient must be observed carefully for signs of toxicity as lactic acid along with the local anaesthetic solution previously confined to the limb is now allowed to wash into the circulatory system within the core (Potter and Perry, 2005; Simpson and Popat, 2002).

Local anaesthesia

The rationale for the administration of local anaesthesia preoperatively is blockage of peripheral sensory nerve stimuli at their very origin, thus abolishing both pain and touch sensation at the operative site. Both subcutaneous and intracutaneous infiltration of the area using a local anaesthetic agent, such as lidocaine or bupivacaine, provide excellent results intra-operatively, though surgeons may also use this technique at completion of the operation to provide immediate postoperative pain relief. Local anaesthesia is eminently suited to many minor procedures undertaken within an ambulatory unit (e.g. anterior eye and skin procedures) and topical application of an anaesthetic agent will desensitise respiratory passages, mucous membranes and the skin surface. A topical anaesthetic ointment is frequently used to 'numb' the back of the hand before gaining intravenous access (Phillips, 2004; Potter and Perry, 2005).

Opportunity for the student

Find out which topical anaesthetic agents are used in your placement area.

Conscious sedation

Conscious sedation is utilised in circumstances where a depressed level of consciousness is needed, rather than complete anaesthesia. Conscious sedation usually involves administration of regional or local anaesthesia to facilitate surgery, in combination with a sedative which causes the patient to relax and sleep. Although conscious sedation is usually undertaken as a planned procedure, it can also prove useful where the operation commences under regional or local anaesthesia (e.g. inguinal hernia repair), but the patient finds the procedure distressing. Further infiltration of the area with the anaesthetic agent in combination with a sedative allows the patient to tolerate the procedure whilst remaining able to respond to verbal command, tactile stimulation and to maintain his/her own airway (DeLamar, 2003; Potter and Perry, 2005).

Opportunity for the student

A booklet produced by BADS (2004c) documents the pathway for patients requiring laparoscopic cholecystectomy, from selection for suitability for day surgery, right through to discharge. Care needs are dealt with comprehensively at each stage of the perioperative journey. Access this information at http://www.daysurgeryuk.org/content/Professionals/BADS-Handbooks.asp and select 'Day Case Laparoscopic Cholecystectomy'.
   Answer the following critical review questions:

- Which anaesthetic technique is used for laparoscopic cholecystectomy?
- An ERCP may be performed as an investigative test for some patients needing removal of their gall bladder. What is an ERCP and what is the indication for this test?

Intra-operative care of the patient

Staff working within the perioperative setting will have a clear understanding of their role within the day surgery unit and the importance of adhering to standards, principles and local and national guidelines. Adherence to standards is a fundamental component of the quality assurance process and will ensure that clinical governance requirements are met. The AfPP produced standards and recommendations which are generally viewed as benchmarks for the standard of care expected within operating theatres (Beesley and Pirie, 2004). Some of the responsibilities of theatre practitioners are outlined below and those new to the clinical environment should observe the care which is delivered in theatre and take full advantage of the numerous learning opportunities which present themselves.

- Positioning the patient
  Under normal circumstances, the body's defence mechanisms protect against undue stretching of ligaments, muscles and the placing of excessive strain on a joint. Anaesthesia abolishes all such protective mechanisms. It may be necessary to place the patient in an unusual position to facilitate surgery; therefore, care must be taken that limbs are kept in correct alignment with extremities and bony prominences protected. Padded supports are used to prevent arms falling from the table, silicone gel pads protect against pressure area damage and nerves (particularly the ulnar nerve) are protected from compression damage (Potter and Perry, 2005).
  The most commonly adopted positions for surgery include:
  - Supine (flat on back)
  - Prone (on front, with head to one side, used for spinal procedures)
  - Lateral (on right or left side, facilitates hip, kidney and thoracic operations)
  - Lithotomy (supine with elevation of legs in stirrups or leg supports, for gynaecological, urological or lower bowel/anal procedures)
  - Trendelenberg (supine with head down tilt. Gravity causes abdominal contents to move towards the diaphragm, thus facilitating the view of gynaecological organs and the pelvis)
  - Reverse Trendelenberg (supine with head-up tilt, useful for upper abdominal procedures and head-and-neck operations) (Smith, 2005)
- Prepping and draping/maintenance of the sterile field
  The surgical site is 'prepped' with an antiseptic solution (povidone-iodine or chlorhexidine gluconate), with the aim of reducing the number of micro-organisms on the skin surface. Gram-negative and gram-positive bacteria, fungi and viruses all increase the potential for development of postoperative wound infections (Beesley and Pirie, 2004). Surgical drapes are then placed immediately around the prepped area. The extent to which the patient is covered with drapes will depend on the type of operation undertaken, e.g. a patient undergoing a laparoscopic cholecystectomy will be completely shrouded in drapes, whilst removal of a tiny skin lesion from the forehead will necessitate minimal draping of the surrounding area.
  Part 3 of EN13795, the standard related to the manufacture of sterile drapes, entered national legislation in 2007, alongside Parts 1 and 2 (Molynyke Health

Care, 2006). This standard has recently been ratified by the British Standards Institute and harmonised by all European Union (EU) countries. The stringent standards outlined in EN13795 will impact on usage of reusable fabric drapes, which is already in decline. Disposable non-woven fabrics have excellent liquid resistance, tensile strength and *hydrophobic* properties and are, therefore, highly suitable for surgical drapes and gowns.

Sterile drapes covering the patient, those draping essential equipment which cannot be sterilised and those used to cover the instrument trolley(s) prior to the laying out of instruments together constitute the 'sterile field'. Non-'scrubbed' personnel in theatre must navigate around this delineated area (not between the operating table and instrument trolley) and every effort must be made to avoid contamination of the sterile field.

- The 'scrub' role

The scrub practitioner is responsible for supervising the patient's intra-operative care and will act as patient advocate if the need arises. Privacy and dignity of the patient will be ensured at all times. Prior to commencement of the list, he/she will ensure that all instrumentation is present, equipment is functioning correctly and the theatre is well stocked. The scrub practitioner will not allow commencement of any procedure until he/she has seen the patient's consent form and been informed of any allergies or prostheses. During the operation, and using an aseptic technique, the scrub practitioner will provide skilled assistance to the surgeon, handling instrumentation and medical devices, whilst at the same time conducting 'counts' of instruments and sundry items, such as swabs, hypodermic needles, blades and atraumatic sutures. 'Counting in' of instruments and sundry items occurs prior to commencement of the procedure and as additional equipment is needed intra-operatively. Items are also documented within the patient's ICP and on the theatre whiteboard. Towards termination of the procedure and commencing with closure of any body cavity, three full checks of all instruments and sundry items will occur. This ensures that all medical devices are accounted for.

The challenge of delivering health care within the UK has necessitated changes in recent times, resulting largely from introduction of European Working Time Regulations in 1998. Drastic reductions in the working hours of junior doctors has already had a profound effect on attendance within day surgery units and as the European Working Time Directive becomes mandatory in 2009, the absence of junior doctors will leave a considerable skills gap (Gindill, 2007). To meet the needs of patients and the service, perioperative practitioners are now encouraged to extend their scope of practice and act as first assistant to the surgeon. To a degree, informal 'assisting' the surgeon has been common practice for many years, but 'dual rolling' (assisting the surgeon with the operation whilst at the same time looking after instruments and counts) is not viewed as good practice. In light of this, the Perioperative Care Collaborative (2003) highlighted the need for perioperative practitioners to be aware of the legal and ethical implications of working outside their scope of practice and defined new roles involving further competency-based training.

Exciting opportunities for role development therefore exist within the theatre environment as Advanced Scrub Practitioners (ASPs), now deemed to be 'expert' practitioners, who are able to replace medical staff assisting at the operating table.

The advent of the Surgical Care Practitioner (SCP) has resulted in practitioners who not only assist with surgery, but are capable of undertaking minor surgical procedures indirectly supervised by a consultant (e.g. circumcisions and herniae repair). SCPs may also conduct their own pre-assessment and follow-up clinics (Royal College of Surgeons of England, 2007).

- Deep vein thrombosis (DVT) prophylaxis

  Immobility on the operating table in combination with the effects of surgery and anaesthesia can predispose the surgical patient towards developing a DVT. Preventative measures include pre- and postoperative injections of anticoagulant therapy (e.g. Clexane), antiembolism stockings and the application of sequential compression devices preoperatively. Intra-operatively, chambers within these leggings inflate and deflate in sequence. Using a recommended pressure of 40 mm Hg, blood is gradually forced back towards the heart reducing the risk of pooling in the deep veins and hence DVT (Smith, 2005).

- Electrosurgery (or diathermy)

  Diathermy is used intra-operatively to coagulate vessels and cut through tissues. The diathermy machine (electrosurgical generator) converts normal mains electricity from 50 Hz to between 500 000 Hz and 1 000 000 Hz. The resulting very high (radio)-frequency current does not excite contractile cells (e.g. the myocardium) because it has low tissue penetration; hence, the ventricular fibrillation normally associated with mains electrocution is avoided (Al-Shaikh and Stacey, 2002).

  A choice of monopolar and bipolar instruments are available for surgery. When monopolar diathermy is used, an electrical circuit is created in which the patient's body forms a significant element of the electrical pathway. Current flows from the generator, through a diathermy lead, into the active electrode (surgeon's instrument). Current density is high because it is channelled through the tips of instruments which are very small. When applied to the patient, the innate resistance encountered as the current attempts to pass through tissues causes a rise in temperature.

  The heat generated can be used by the surgeon to cut, or coagulate tissues, depending on the type of active electrode utilised. The current then continues through the patient's body, is attracted to the return electrode (a diathermy plate attached to the skin surface) and is returned to the generator. Heat is not generated at the return electrode because it has a relatively large surface area in comparison with the active electrode and therefore a low current density (Wicker and O'Neil, 2006).

  Bipolar electrosurgery works at lower power settings and is less invasive since it combines both active and return electrodes within the surgical instrument itself (forceps or scissors). The current passes between the tips of the instrument and the tissues contained therein and does *not* pass through the patient's body. Hence, a diathermy plate is unnecessary. In day surgery, bipolar is particularly suitable for children, mucous membranes (eyes and lips), extremities (fingers and foreskin), skin tissues and in situations where the patient has an older type of pacemaker in situ.

- The role of the 'circulator'

  The 'circulator' or 'runner' will assist in the preparation of the theatre environment and will help anaesthetic personnel position the patient correctly for surgery.

Other important tasks include application of sequential compression devices, a diathermy plate and shaving of the operative site (if these are deemed necessary). The circulator will supply the 'sterile' scrub practitioner with sterile items and additional instrumentation required intra-operatively will document the care delivered within the integrated care plan, pass on messages, pot specimens and complete histology and microbiology request forms.

- Infected cases
  It is usual to undertake infected cases at the end of the list to reduce the risk of transmission of disease and allow for terminal cleaning of the theatre.
- Health and safety issues
  Within a day surgery unit, throughput of patients can be rapid. It is essential therefore to establish:
  - Correct consent
  - Correct operative site
  - Safe transfer and positioning
  - Prevention of diathermy burns
  - Correct counts
  - Completed documentation
  - Effective infection control policies and procedures

Recovery and post-anaesthetic considerations

- Function of the recovery room/patient handover
  A day surgery recovery unit provides a dedicated, calm and therapeutic environment in which patients are closely monitored until such time as deemed fit to return to the ward. The recovery practitioner will monitor baseline observations and continually assess the condition and individual needs of the patient, providing therapeutic intervention as necessary.

  The anaesthetist, anaesthetic practitioner and, ideally, the scrub practitioner will accompany the patient into recovery. Effective communication between theatre staff and the recovery practitioner is essential. Handover should include the following information regarding the patient:
  - Name
  - Type of operation performed
  - Allergies/medical condition
  - Mode of anaesthesia
  - Condition intra-operatively
  - Untoward anaesthetic or surgical events, e.g. haemorrhage
  - Analgesia/muscle relaxants/antibiotics administered
  - Intravenous fluids (with further regime prescribed if necessary)
  - Type of wound closure and dressing
  - Infiltration of the wound with local anaesthetic
  - Site of drains/catheters
  - Discharge pain relief should be written up
- Emergence from anaesthesia/elimination of anaesthetic agents from the body
  Due to the short-term nature of anaesthesia administered within day surgery, patients will frequently regain consciousness in theatre. If 'emergence' from

anaesthesia has not occurred prior to entry to recovery, protection and support of the patient's airway is the first priority and one-to-one care is essential. Patients must be breathing adequately and able to maintain their own airway before any form of breathing tube is removed (Wicker and O'Neil, 2006).

Anaesthetic drugs are removed from the body by a process called *elimination*, so-called because normal homeostatic processes commence elimination of drugs from the bloodstream by breaking them down within various organs. A few drugs, e.g. volatile agents, are not altered within the body and exit by the same route as they were administered, via the lungs. Most drugs, however, undergo chemical alteration (metabolism) prior to elimination which breaks down the drug into a molecule easier to eliminate. For example metabolism will convert a drug which is highly lipid (fat) soluble into metabolites (compounds) which are water soluble. In the process, the biological activity of the administered drug is reduced or abolished, though some resulting metabolites may still have remaining biological activity (Whelan, 2000; Wicker and O'Neil, 2006).

The liver is the site of breakdown for most drugs and two types of chemical reactions termed Phase 1 and Phase 2 achieve this. Phase 1 involves an enzyme system called cytochrome P-450, which can bring about a variety of changes to the drug molecule including oxidation, but ultimately the remaining molecule remains detached. Phase 2 reactions have their effect by then reacting with the detached molecule produced by Phase 1 and, in a process called 'conjugation', combine it with another, resulting in a molecule larger in size, more water soluble and therefore more easily eliminated. Certain drugs however, bypass Phase 1 completely and are broken down only by Phase 2 reactions (Whelan, 2000).

In addition to breakdown within the liver, a minority of drugs may be metabolised within the kidney, lungs, plasma or intestines. Most metabolites, along with a minority of drugs which are not themselves broken down, are subsequently eliminated in the urine (smaller molecules) and/or bile (larger molecules). Within the kidney, elimination occurs because molecules are:

(a)   Filtered into the glomerulus passively
(b)   Secreted from the proximal renal tubule
(c)   Diffused out from the distal renal tubule

Elimination via bile occurs because liver cells actively secrete metabolites into bile (Whelan, 2000).
- Patient monitoring
  Constant surveillance of the patient is essential with the aim of pre-empting postoperative complications such as laryngospasm, respiratory distress/obstruction and cardiac arrhythmia. Five- to ten-minute observations of the following are noted and recorded within the integrated care plan:
  - Breathing rate
  - Blood pressure
  - Pulse rate
  - Oxygen saturation levels
  - Oozing from wound/drain site

The patient is also monitored for signs of pain and PONV. While some patients will require little in the way of pain relief, certain operations such as laparoscopic cholecystectomy may cause both pain and nausea. In this instance a 'multi-modal' approach to pain is taken because non-steroidal anti-inflammatory drugs and a local anaesthetic in combination with opioids allow considerable reduction in the amount of opioid administered. This facilitates a speedy recovery with reduction in the nausea associated with opioid use. If nausea does occur then ondansetron or dexamethasone would provide suitable therapy (BADS, 2004c).

On average, day surgery patients remain in recovery for 30 min. Once vital signs are stable, the patient is oriented to preoperative levels and remaining discharge criteria are met, then *first-stage recovery* is complete and the patient may return to the ward (McEwen, 2003). A comprehensive handover between the recovery practitioner and ward nurse is essential. In addition to relaying information which accompanied the patient from theatre, the ward nurse is furnished with an account of the patient's progress in recovery.

Discharge from the day surgery unit

Second-stage recovery commences back on the ward and when an appropriately qualified person deems the patient to be sufficiently recovered, then discharge takes place (McEwen, 2003). The practitioner discharging the patient from the ward should ensure:

- Vital signs are stable.
- Clear fluids are tolerated, particularly diabetic/nauseated patients.
- Micturition has occurred.
- Orientation has returned to previous levels.
- There is no untoward bleeding/oozing from wound.
- Pain is controlled.
- Take-home analgesia is dispensed.
- Mobilisation (dependent on procedure) has occurred and mobility aids supplied.
- Escort with private transport is in attendance.
- Close supervision is available for 24 hours postoperatively.
- Follow-up appointment/community care are arranged if required.
- Post-discharge instructions and expectations are clarified.
- An emergency contact number is supplied (Beesley and Pirie, 2004; McMillan, 2005).

An unplanned overnight admission will prove necessary in the event the patient returns late from theatre, since inadequate time will be available for recovery. Likewise, when the extent of surgery is greater than originally planned, where complications such as bleeding, PONV or poor pain management occur. Procedures to deal with unplanned admissions need to be in place and these must be recorded and audited (NHS Modernisation Agency, 2005). Discharged patients receive a follow-up telephone call the following day to check on progress and provide reassurance (DH, 2002; McMillan, 2005).

> **Scenario**
> Mrs Green has been referred to the day surgery unit for guide-wire excision of an impalpable breast lesion. The patient is naturally anxious about the procedure and is experiencing some discomfort from the localisation wire which was inserted under image intensification in the radiology department earlier in the day.
>
> (1) In this situation, the student nurse working within the day surgery unit can do much to help Mrs Green. Which skills can be employed here?
> (2) A diathermy hand-switching pencil will generally be utilised to excise the breast tissue surrounding the wire. Investigate the means by which this device works and its advantages when compared with a scalpel blade.
> (3) Once excised, the lesion (still containing the wire) will be examined within the X-ray department and in the event excision of the lesion is thought to be complete, the specimen will be transferred into a specimen pot. Which preserving solution is used to cover the specimen prior to its transfer for histological examination and what is the relevance of documentation here?

Summary

A brief overview of the patient's perioperative journey has been outlined here, from admission, through surgery, to discharge. A comprehensive and detailed analysis of the work of the perioperative practitioner is beyond the scope of this chapter; however, it is hoped the reader will have gained some insight into life behind the scenes of the day surgery ward and theatre environment. Opportunities for role development for both nurses and ODPs are currently at an exciting stage. The student should therefore be proactive in seeking opportunities to follow patients through their surgical episode in order that this challenging, exciting and rewarding environment can be experienced.

Glossary of terms

Anaesthesia
A loss of bodily feeling and sensation with or without loss of consciousness

Analgesia
Commonly referred to as a 'painkiller' from the Greek *an-* 'without' and *-algia*, 'pain'

Hydrophobic
With water-resistant qualities

Narcosis
The unconsciousness induced by narcotic medication

References

Al-Shaikh, B. and Stacey, S. (2002) *Essentials of Anaesthetic Equipment*, 2nd ed. London: Churchill Livingstone.

American Society of Anesthesiologists (1999) Practice guidelines for preoperative fasting and the use of pharmacologic agents to reduce the risk of pulmonary aspiration: application to healthy patients undergoing elective procedures. *Anesthesiology* 90(3), pp. 896–905.

Beauchamp, T. and Childress, J. (2001) *Principles of Biomedical Ethics*, 5th ed. Oxford: Oxford University Press.

Beesley, J. and Pirie, S. (eds) (2004) *NATN Standards and Recommendations for Safe Perioperative Practice.* Harrogate: National Association of Theatre Nurses.

British Association of Day Surgery (BADS) (2003) *Commissioning Day Surgery.* Available from: www.bads.co.uk (accessed 14 June 2007).

British Association of Day Surgery (BADS) (2004a) *Integrated Care Pathways for Day Surgery Patients.* Available from: http://www.daysurgeryuk.org/content/Professionals/ BADS-Handbooks.asp (accessed 14 June 2007).

British Association of Day Surgery (BADS) (2004b) *Spinal Anaesthesia: A Practical Guide.* Available from: http://www.daysurgeryuk.org/content/Professionals/BADS-Handbooks.asp (accessed 14 June 2007).

British Association of Day Surgery (BADS) (2004c) *Day Case Laparoscopic Cholecystectomy.* Available from: http://www.daysurgeryuk.org/content/Professionals/BADS-Handbooks.asp (accessed 14 June 2007).

DeLamar, L. (2003) Anesthesia, in Rothrock, J. (ed.) *Alexander's Care of the Patient in Surgery*, 12th ed. USA: Mosby, pp. 219–251.

Department of Health (DH) (2002) *Day Surgery: Operational Guide.* UK: Department of Health Publications.

Department of Health (DH) (2005) *Treatment Centres: Delivering Faster, Quality Care and Choice for NHS Patients.* Available from: http://www.dh.gov.uk/en/ Publicationsandstatistics/Publications/PublicationsPolicyAndGuidance/DH_4100523 (accessed 1 May 2007).

Department of Health (DH) (2007a) *Saws and Scalpels to Lasers and Robots: Advances in Surgery. Clinical Case for Change: Report by Professor Sir Ara Darzi.* Available from: http://www.dh.gov.uk/en/Publicationsandstatistics/Publications/PublicationsPolicyAnd Guidance/DH_073904 (accessed 31 May 2007).

Department of Health (DH) (2007b) *Consent Key Documents.* Available from: http://www.dh.gov.uk/en/Policyandguidance/Healthandsocialcaretopics/Consent /Consentgeneralinformation/index.htm (accessed 1 June 2007).

General Medical Council (2006) *Seeking Patients' Consent: The Ethical Considerations.* Available from: http://www.gmc-uk.org/guidance/current/library/consent.asp#reviewing (accessed 1 June 2007).

Gindill, J. (2007) The multi-skilled day surgery practitioner. *Journal of Perioperative Practice* 17(9), pp. 437–440.

Griffiths, R. (2000) Anaesthetic drugs, in *Back to Basics-Perioperative Practice Principles.* UK: National Association of Theatre Nurses, pp. 30–33.

Ince, C., Skinner, A. and Taft, E. (2000) Scientific principles in relation to the anaesthetic machine, in Davy, A. and Ince, S. (eds) *Fundamentals of Operating Department Practice.* London: Greenwich Medical Media Ltd, pp. 75–97.

McEwen, D. (2003) Ambulatory surgery, in Rothrock, J (ed.). *Alexander's Care of the Patient in Surgery*, 12th ed. USA: Mosby, pp. 1189–1210.

McMillan, R. (2005) Day surgery, in Woodhead, K. and Whicker, P. (eds) *A Textbook of Perioperative Care.* London: Elsevier Churchill Livingstone, pp. 199–220.

McNeil, B. (2005) Malignant hyperthermia. *British Journal of Perioperative Nursing* 15(9), pp. 376–382.

Molynyke Health Care (2006) *New European Standard – The Final Countdown.* Available from: http://www.thestandard.molnlycke.com/item.asp?id=24505&si=67 (accessed 23 June 2007).

National Patient Safety Agency (NPSA) (2007) *Putting Patient Safety First*. Available from: http://www.npsa.nhs.uk/patientsafety/alerts-and-directives/notices/wristbands/ (accessed 3 September 2007).

NHS Modernisation Agency (2002) *National Good Practice Guidance on Preoperative Assessment for Day Surgery*. Available from: http://www.cancerimprovement.nhs.uk/ %5Cdocuments%5CPublications%20from%20NHS%20Modernisation%20Agency% 5CPreoperative%20guidance%20for%20daycase%20surgery.pdf (accessed 23 June 2007).

NHS Moderrisation Agency (2005) Day Surgery. A Good Practice Guide Available from: http://www.wise.nhs.uk/cmsWISE/Cross+Cutting+Themes/access/elective/documents/ documents.htm (accessed 20 June 2007).

Perioperative Care Collaborative (August 2003) The provision of the non-medical perioperative practitioner working as first assistant to the surgeon. A position statement. *British Journal of Perioperative Nursing – Supplement 13*(8), pp. 1–4.

Phillips, N. (2004) *Berry and Kohn's Operating Room Technique*, 10th ed. USA: Mosby.

Potter, P. and Perry, A. (2005) *Fundamentals of Nursing*, 6th ed. USA: Elsevier Mosby.

Pyrek, K. (2007) *Pre-op Prep Should Safeguard Skin Integrity*. Available from: http://www.infectioncontroltoday.com/articles/231topics.html (accessed 7 June 2007).

Rogan Foy, C. and Timmins, F. (2004) Improving communication in day surgery settings. *Nursing Standard 19*(7), pp. 37–42.

Royal College of Nursing (2004) *Children/Young People in Day Surgery*. Available from: http://www.rcn.org.uk/publications/pdf/daysurgery_cyp.pdf (accessed 13 June 2007).

Simpson, P. and Popat, M. (2002) *Understanding Anaesthesia*, 4th ed. London: Butterworth Heinneman.

Smith, C. (2005) Care of the patient undergoing surgery, in Woodhead, K. and Wicker, P. (eds) *A Textbook of Perioperative Care*. China: Elsevier, pp. 161–180.

StaffNurse.com (2007) *Patient Wristbands to be Standardised*. Available from: http://www.staffnurse.com/nursing-news-articles/patient-wristbands-to-be-standardised-2545.html (accessed 2 September 2007).

Tanner, J., Woodings, D. and Moncaster, K. (2006) Preoperative hair removal to reduce surgical site infection. *The Cochrane Collaboration*, Art. No: CD004122. DOI: 10.1002/14651858.CD004122.pub3 [online]. Available from: http://www.cochrane.org/ reviews/en/ab004122.html (accessed 7 June 2007).

The Royal College of Surgeons of England (2007) *What Are Surgical Care Practitioners?* Available from: http://www.rcseng.ac.uk/career/nonmed/whatarescps.html (accessed 13 June 2007).

Whelan, E. (2000) Pharmacological principles of drug administration, in Davy, A. and Ince, S. (eds) *Fundamentals of Operating Department Practice*. London. Greenwich Medical Media Ltd, pp. 133–139.

Whelan, E. and Davies, H. (2000) The pharmacology of drugs used in general anaesthesia, in Davy, A. and Ince, S. (eds) *Fundamentals of Operating Department Practice*. London: Greenwich Medical Media Ltd, pp. 141–158.

Wicker, P. and O'Neil, J. (2006) *Caring for the Perioperative Patient*. Oxford: Blackwell Publishing.

World Health Organization (2006) *Blood Safety and Clinical Technology-Guidelines on Prevention and Control of Hospital Associated Infections*. Available from: http://www.searo.who.int/EN/Section10/Section17/Section53/Section362_1115.htm (accessed 7 June 2007).

Chapter 10

Renal nursing

Peter Ellis

Learning objectives

(1) Describe what happens to patients when the kidneys are damaged
(2) Identify the nature, purpose and differences between renal outpatient services
(3) Define the monitoring, management and treatment roles of the nurse within the outpatient areas as well as the scope for professional development
(4) Consider health education and health promotion strategies, opportunities, barriers and threats

---

Introduction

Definition

Renal outpatients provide care for individuals with various stages and types of renal disease. These will include people with chronic kidney disease (CKD), established renal failure (ERF) and recovering acute renal failure (ARF). Some outpatient areas deal with single, renal-related problems, like the renal anaemia clinic.

Working in renal care offers a wide variety of opportunities. The care of the renal patient ranges from community-based screening and management of early renal disease through inpatient care, chronic and acute dialysis, transplant and ultimately palliative and terminal care. This variety means that the renal practitioner is presented with a myriad of choices as to where to practice and exercise both their chronic and acute nursing skills.

Another positive aspect of renal care is the opportunity to work in a diverse, yet close-knit, inter-professional team. Many renal units have a dedicated team of professionals, including social workers, counsellors, occupational therapists, nurses, dialysis technicians, doctors and physiotherapists, whose expertise helps maximise the quality of the patient experience.

For the nurse working in renal care there are many outpatient areas in which to practice. The purpose of these areas and the role of the nurse providing high-quality care to the patient population are described in this chapter, as are some opportunities for advanced and innovative practice.

In 2004 the first renal National Service Framework (NSF) presented the renal community with a number of new challenging standards. This NSF is entitled 'Part One: Dialysis and Transplantation' and most of the target standards allude to increasing patient choice and communication (Department of Health (DH), 2004). These themes are reflected in the quality requirements of 'Part Two: Chronic Kidney Disease, Acute Renal Failure and End of Life Care' (DH, 2005).

Opportunity for the student

Visit the British Department of Health website and download the renal NSFs and read the executive summaries.

This chapter starts by explaining some basic functions of the kidney, the causes, effects and classifications of CKD and some of the specific investigations (e.g. renal ultrasound) and tests (e.g. blood tests) which are undertaken. The second half will explore the role of the practitioner in the various renal outpatient departments. Throughout the chapter reference will be made to ideas and themes highlighted and explored elsewhere in this book and opportunities for learning and reflection will be identified.

Functions of the kidney

The main function of the kidneys is to excrete the waste products of metabolism and to control the levels of electrolytes and water within the body. The kidneys also play an important role in the regulation of blood pressure, calcium metabolism and the production of erythrocytes (Box 10.1).

Checkpoint

Revise your knowledge of the functions of the kidney.

Box 10.1 Functions of the kidney

Functions of the kidney
- Excretory
  - Waste products of metabolism (namely creatinine and urea)
- Regulatory
  - Water volume
  - Water osmolality
  - Electrolyte balance
  - Acid–base balance
- Metabolic
  - Activation of vitamin D
  - Production of renin
  - Production of erythropoietin

The classifications of renal disease: renal disease may take any of three main forms:

- Acute: characterised by a rapid onset followed by recovery over a short period of time
- Chronic: a permanent, normally progressive deterioration in renal function
- Established: advanced stage of chronic renal failure which would result in death if some form of dialysis or transplant is not undertaken

ARF is often seen in the elderly and normally results from some incident in which the body becomes dehydrated, as in severe diarrhoea and vomiting or trauma. Other causes may include surgery, especially where the aorta is cross clamped or where the heart is stopped, e.g. coronary artery bypass (Stein et al., 2004). ARF is invariably managed as an inpatient episode.

CKD has many causes (see next section). The prevalence of CKD is hard to quantify as many individuals have CKD but die of something else, perhaps renal-related, before it is diagnosed (Khan et al., 1994). Interestingly, the incidence and prevalence of known CKD is increasing, perhaps as a result of screening initiatives and in relation to the increasing age of the population and the rise in other chronic diseases that may cause CKD, e.g. diabetes. People with CKD are generally managed as outpatients or even by their general practitioner. People with mild-to-moderate CKD may be seen in the general nephrology clinic and those with more advanced disease are seen in a multidisciplinary clinic in the low-clearance (sometimes called the pre-dialysis or advanced kidney care) clinic (LCC).

ERF, also known as end-stage renal failure or disease, is increasing in incidence and prevalence. The UK Renal Registry figures show that the number of people on haemodialysis at the end of 2005 was 17 645, the number on peritoneal dialysis was 5057 and the number with a functioning transplant was 19 074 (UK Renal Registry, 2006). The number of adults in the UK accepted for dialysis or transplantation in 2005 was 6485, representing an acceptance rate of 108 persons per million of population (UK Renal Registry, 2006).

Table 10.1 Important causes of CKD in the UK

Diagnosis	Description
Cause uncertain	Often the result of late referral, so the kidneys are too shrunken to biopsy
Diabetic nephropathy	A result of blood vessel damage caused by high blood sugars
Glomerulonephritis	Inflammation of the kidney either autoimmune or as a result of infection
Pyelonephritis	Infection of the kidneys, or ureters, often the result of backflow of infected urine from the bladder
Renovascular disease	Occurs when one or both of the arteries supplying the kidneys is partially or totally occluded
Polycystic kidney disease	Is a genetic disease which has a dominant pattern of inheritance
Hypertensive kidney disease	The result of increased pressure on the small blood vessels in the kidneys

People with ERF (people on dialysis or with a transplant) are generally managed as outpatients visiting the hospital either three times a week as a haemodialysis patient or as little as twice a year following successful transplantation.

The causes of chronic kidney disease

There are a large number of potential causes of CKD. Any one patient may have more than one cause and in some instances the exact cause of their CKD is never known. Table 10.1 lists the main causes of ERF in adults new to dialysis, or transplantation, in 2005 as identified by the UK Renal Registry (2006).

The signs and symptoms of chronic kidney disease

The signs and symptoms of CKD are strongly related to the functions of the kidneys and severity of the disease. Many individuals with CKD do not know they have it until it is quite advanced; others have their disease diagnosed at an early stage, perhaps when they are attending a clinic for other associated conditions like diabetes or hypertension.

The symptoms of renal disease are often described as being insidious and are easily mistaken for the signs of aging. Common signs and symptoms of renal disease include:

- Lethargy – associated with poor dietary intake, breathlessness and anaemia
- Anorexia – which is a lack of appetite associated with gastrointestinal tract disturbance and proteinuria
- Shortness of breath – as a result of acidosis, anaemia and pulmonary oedema and effusions

- Peripheral and pulmonary oedema – as a result of hypoalbuminaemia and inability to excrete water
- Hypertension – which is both a cause and an effect of CKD and may be exacerbated by inability to regulate body water levels
- Proteinuria – as a result of damage to the glomerular basement membrane
- Haematuria – as a result of damage to the glomerular basement membrane
- Anaemia – from occult and iatrogenic blood loss and lack of erythropoietin
- Raised serum creatinine and urea – as the kidneys fail to excrete the waste products of protein metabolism
  (Levy et al., 2006)

Opportunity for the student

Spend some time with a renal patient and discuss the signs and symptoms of renal disease that caused them to seek help.

Renal investigations and tests

Quite simply, the presence of CKD is established through a simple blood test which detects raised levels of serum creatinine and urea. Urea alone, however, is a poor marker of renal function being strongly affected by the hydration levels and diet (Levy et al., 2006; Mahon and Hattersley, 2002). Creatinine may also be misleading as an individual may lose up to 50% of their renal function and still have a reading within normal limits (Mahon and Hattersley, 2002). It is now common practice to estimate renal function from a calculation based on an individual's age, gender and serum creatinine. Such a calculation gives an estimated glomerular filtration rate (eGFR) a more accurate representation of renal function (Levy et al., 2006).

Opportunity for the student

Find out what, in health, a normal GFR is and its units of measurement.

An eGFR does not, however, give any clues as to the cause of the kidney disease. The cause of the kidney disease is established by determining the patient's medical, family and social history, and clinical examination and the application of further tests.

Various clues as to the aetiology of the kidney disease may be gained by establishing whether the individual has a history of other chronic diseases which may affect the kidneys, including diabetes, hypertension or prostate disease. In other cases treatments for medical conditions which may affect the kidneys may be evident, e.g. the long-term use of non-steroidal anti-inflammatory drugs for disease like rheumatoid arthritis or use of immunosupressives, for example, following heart or lung transplant.

Familial history taking may uncover a family history of renal disease (polycystic kidneys being the most common); social history may point to the potential for infection with human immunodeficiency virus (HIV) (associated with HIV nephropathy) or hepatitis. Some disease may be readily obvious on initial examination, such as retinopathy associated with previously undiagnosed diabetes.

As with all diagnostic testing the tests used to establish the cause of kidney disease are escalated up from the most simple, cheap, safe and non-invasive to tests which are more complicated to undertake, are more expensive, have some inherent risk attached and are invasive. Simple tests include:

- Urinalysis
- Albumin (or protein) to creatinine ratio
- Blood tests for autoantibodies
- Kidney ureter and bladder ultrasound
- Doppler ultrasound

More sophisticated investigations include:

- Computerised tomography (CT)
- Magnetic resonance imaging (MRI)
- Radionucleotide imaging
- Renal angiography
- Renal biopsy

Cumulative knowledge

Find out how these investigations work and what they tell the health care team. You will find some answers in Chapter 7.

Urinalysis

The presence of blood and protein in the urine (haematuria and proteinuria) do not indicate the cause of renal disease, but they may demonstrate the presence of renal disease (Terrill, 2002). Haematuria is commonly associated with the presence of infection, or malignant disease, in the urinary tract (Levy et al., 2006).

Proteinuria may indicate disease in any part of the urinary tract and is associated with damage to the glomerulus or the renal tubules. A significant cause of proteinuria is urinary tract infection and should be excluded early on (Levy et al., 2006).

Albumin (protein)-to-creatinine ratio

It is often useful to quantify the amount of protein in the urine, as levels in excess of 1 g/day will require further investigation. Twenty-four-hour urine collections are unreliable due to timing issues and forgetfulness and have largely been superseded by a spot check of urine where the ratio of creatinine to protein in the urine is calculated. The protein-to-creatinine ratio correlates well with 24-hour protein excretion with a ratio of 1 (conventional units) or 120 mg/mmol (SI units) equating to 1 g of protein excreted per 24 hour (Levy et al., 2006).

Blood tests for autoantibodies

Some diseases result from the immune system attacking cells within the body; specific blood tests can detect if the immune system has created antibodies to specific renal cells.

Kidney ureter and bladder ultrasound

This is an efficient and non-invasive way of diagnosing, or excluding, many causes of renal failure. Principal signs of renal disease which may indicate the cause of the CKD and may be detected using ultrasound include:

- The presence/absence of cysts
- Evidence of outflow obstruction (incomplete bladder emptying and smooth-edged renal calyces)
- Kidney size (in health, the kidneys are roughly 11 cm pole to pole, and in chronic renal disease they are usually shrunken or hypertrophied)
- Kidney density (the chronically damaged or hypertrophied kidney is more echo bright and appears more white than the healthy kidney)

Cumulative knowledge

Revisit Chapter 7 to remind yourself about how ultrasound works.

Doppler ultrasound

Doppler ultrasound is useful in detecting renal artery stenosis (narrowing) or the presence of a thrombus (clot). Doppler detects the flow of blood through major vessels in the body by examining how sound waves bounce off of moving objects, like blood (Medlineplus, 2007).

Computerised tomography

CT uses X-rays to create cross-sectional pictures of the kidneys, bladder and ureters and may be useful in the diagnosis of diseases which affect the anatomy of the kidney or urinary system (Medlineplus, 2007).

Magnetic resonance imaging

Like the CT scan, the MRI is excellent for viewing microanatomy as well as defining renal lesions. The MRI scanner uses powerful magnets to line up the hydrogen atoms in the body in a certain way, radio waves are then sent into the body and the machine records the ways in which different tissues respond to these (see Chapter 7 for more detail).

Radionucleotide imaging

Radionucleotide imaging is used where there are questions about the functioning of the kidneys. It may be used to examine for diseases of the blood vessels and can be used to quantify renal function. A small amount of a radioactive substance is injected intravenously and its progression through the blood vessels of the kidney is monitored.

Renal angiography

Renal angiography provides the best method for detecting renovascular disorders, in particular problems associated with the renal artery, as well as signs of trauma or tumours; it also provides an opportunity for interventions like the positioning of stents. Radiopaque dye is injected into the renal arteries via a catheter inserted into the femoral artery.

Renal biopsy

Renal biopsy may be regarded as the definitive method of diagnosing the cause of CKD, especially different forms of glomerulonephritis, other glomerular disorders and interstitial nephritis. Renal biopsies are undertaken using ultrasound to identify the position of the kidney and are always done as an inpatient admission as the patient will need 24-hour bed rest. The biopsy samples tissue from the kidney medulla and glomerular apparatus, in particular, and is checked under a microscope by laboratory technicians to ensure that an adequate sample has been achieved before the procedure is completed.

Areas of care

The areas within the renal department reflect the wide variety of work that the different classification of renal disease give rise to. These include infrequent contact in the nephrology outpatient setting right through to the high-dependency-ward setting where people with ARF are cared for (Box 10.2).

Box 10.2 Areas within the renal department

Inpatient renal areas

   Most wards are a mix of high and low dependency and include patients admitted for medical and surgical care as well as investigations

Outpatient renal areas

   Nephrology outpatients – chronic kidney disease and hypertension management (usually physician led)

   Low-clearance clinic – severe chronic kidney disease approaching established renal failure (often nurse led)

   Anaemia clinic – usually for non-dialysis patients to manage erythropoietin and iron administration (usually nurse led)

   Haemodialysis unit – an outpatient area which is always nurse led

   Peritoneal dialysis clinic – an outpatient area which is always nurse led

   Transplant clinic – where patients are prepared for, and cared, for following a kidney transplant

   Conservative management clinic – where people who decide not to dialyse are cared for

   Access planning clinic – where pro-active decisions about the creation and management of dialysis access are made

Nephrology outpatients

The nephrology outpatients' clinic is the first point of contact for most patients with CKD. The purpose of the clinic is to:

- Establish the cause of the renal disease
- To manage the renal disease
- To manage the signs and symptoms of renal disease

Usually the patient is seen by a physician who may order a number of blood tests, a renal ultrasound, other kidney, ureter and bladder imaging and possibly admission to hospital for a renal biopsy.

Opportunity for the student

What blood tests are undertaken in nephrology outpatients? Why? Discuss these with your mentor.

In the nephrology clinic setting the nurse will often need to undertake urinalysis to look for and quantify the signs of kidney disease. The patient's blood pressure is also taken, as hypertension is both a cause and a sign of renal disease.

Opportunity for the student

An important task in any renal clinic is to weigh the patient. What is the purpose of weighing the patient and specifically what does this show in relation to kidney disease? Discuss this with your mentor.

Low-clearance or the pre-dialysis clinic

The term *low clearance* refers to reduced (or low) creatinine clearance, which is indicative of reduced renal function. With the recent increase in conservative management of ERF (see later) many clinics are now using the name low clearance, or advanced kidney care clinic, as opposed to pre-dialysis clinic to indicate that their purpose is the care of all patients with advanced CKD.

The key roles of the staff in the LCC are to:

- Manage the underlying kidney disease
- Manage the signs and symptoms of advancing kidney disease
- Educate the patient about their condition
- Describe and discuss the options for care with the patient
- Prepare the patient both physically and mentally for life with established renal disease

The role of the inter-professional team is an important one in the LCC as the management of advancing renal disease is complex. Best care for the patient can only be achieved in a holistic manner which embraces all of the expertise of the various renal professionals working together with the patient. Various studies have shown that good preparation for life on dialysis improves the patient's physical, social and mental well-being (Klang et al., 1999; Sesso and Yoshihiro, 1997).

Managing the underlying kidney disease remains an issue even in the LCC as slowing down the progression of the disease means the patient may not need dialysis or a transplant so soon. Methods for slowing down the progression of renal disease depend on the underlying cause but universally include the good management of blood pressure (Ellis and Cairns, 2001).

Signs and symptoms of renal disease are directly related to the functions of the kidney as described earlier in this chapter. The key signs and symptoms that require managing include anaemia, hypertension, fluid balance, breathlessness, renal bone disease and itching.

Opportunity for the student

List the potential causes of breathlessness in the individual with advanced chronic kidney disease.

Renal anaemia clinic

Anaemia is responsible for many of the signs and symptoms of renal disease; these include fatigue, lethargy and breathlessness (Jenkins, 2004). In renal disease the main cause of anaemia is lack of production of the hormone erythropoietin (which stimulates red-blood-cell production and is sometimes referred to as *epo*). The main causes of anaemia associated with kidney disease are:

- Reduced lifespan of erythrocytes as a result of uraemia (down from 120 days)
- Iron, folic acid and vitamin B12 deficiency
- Occult blood loss from the gastrointestinal tract
- Repeated, often unnecessary, blood sampling
- Blood loss in the dialysis circuit

Management of anaemia is generally achieved through supplementation of iron stores, either by tablets or intravenous injection or by the use of erythrocyte-stimulating-agent (ESA) injections.

Nurse specialists run many renal anaemia clinics. The role of the nurse in these clinics is to:

- Order and review appropriate blood tests to identify the cause of the anaemia
- Educate the patient about the causes of renal anaemia and its management and to train the patient to self-administer subcutaneous ESA injections
- Administer intravenous iron injections to provide the 'haem' element of haemoglobin
- To follow up patients receiving ESA therapy to ensure that they achieve the aspirational range of haemoglobin and monitor side effects like hypertension
- To refer on patients with other needs

Current standards for the treatment of renal anaemia, which applies to all patients with CKD, set the aspirational range of haemoglobin (Hb) between 10.5 and 12.5 g/dL with initiation of treatment when the Hb falls below 11 g/dL (National Institute for Health and Clinical Excellence (NHICE), 2006).

Peritoneal dialysis clinic

This is an area which is generally nurse led. Patients cared for in this clinic are trained and supported to complete their own dialysis at home. The most common form of peritoneal dialysis is continuous ambulatory peritoneal dialysis, or CAPD for short, although various automated forms of peritoneal dialysis are in frequent use. Peritoneal dialysis takes advantage of the fact that a semipermeable membrane called the peritoneum lines the abdomen.

Cumulative knowledge

Revise the anatomy and physiology of the peritoneum. What are the names of the two parts of the peritoneal membrane? What, in normal physiology, is the purpose of the peritoneum?

A catheter is inserted into the peritoneal space and is used to instil dialysis fluid (dialysate) which contains none of the waste products of metabolism (urea and creatinine) and physiological levels of important electrolytes like sodium, chloride and magnesium. The fluid contains a strong solution of an osmotic agent (normally glucose) and it also contains a buffer, bicarbonate (or more usually lactate, which is converted into bicarbonate in the liver).

The strong glucose solution exerts an osmotic pressure on the capillary network on the outside of the peritoneum drawing water across the membrane and into the peritoneal space. The waste products of metabolism also cross the membrane into the dialysate this time by diffusion. When diffusion occurs across the membrane it is called dialysis (Graham, 1998).

> **Cumulative knowledge**
>
> Revise osmosis and diffusion, write down a definition and then think about how they help achieve the goals of peritoneal dialysis.

The physiological levels of other electrolytes in the dialysate means that there is no diffusion gradient, so there is a minimal net movement of these electrolytes in either direction.

The role of the nurses in the peritoneal dialysis clinic is the initial and ongoing training and support of patients on peritoneal dialysis (Wild, 2002). The need for educational training and communication skills is fundamental to achieving this goal. The peritoneal dialysis clinic relies on good inter-professional working to achieve maximum independence for the patient, with the dietitian, social worker/care manager and occupational therapists providing valuable input.

The major complications associated with CAPD are:

- Peritonitis, which occurs when infection is introduced into the peritoneal cavity
- Exit-site infection, which occurs at the point on the abdominal wall where the CAPD catheter exits the body
- Technique failure, which occurs as some individuals are unable to learn how to undertake CAPD or are prevented from doing so because of problems like arthritis, poor sight, chronic constipation or some other bowel disorder

The haemodialysis unit

Haemodialysis is quite simply a process by which impurities are removed from the blood by an artificial kidney, or 'dialyser'. Dialysis makes use of the same biological process as peritoneal dialysis, namely diffusion. Dialysis is simply diffusion except a membrane separates the fluids so that some constituents do not mix. Blood is passed through the membrane (hollow fibres) and dialysis fluid (dialysate) passes around the outside. Particles diffuse between the blood and dialysate so that toxins, like urea and creatinine, which enter the dialysate from the blood can be washed away down the drain. Other constituents of blood, like red and white blood cells and platelets, and some proteins are too large to pass through the membrane and are returned to the patient (Ellis, 1997).

The rate and amount of transfer of toxins and important electrolyte is controlled by their concentration in the dialysate. Electrolytes which need to be kept within normal ranges, like potassium, sodium and magnesium, are present in normal concentrations in the dialysate. Toxins which need to be removed from the blood (e.g. creatinine and urea) are not present in the dialysate. Bicarbonate, which is often low in dialysis patients, is present in high concentrations in dialysate and will pass from it into the blood (Ellis, 1997).

Dialysate mainly consists of highly purified water because a dialysis patient's blood is exposed to about 500 mL of water every minute during dialysis that is 120 L during a 4-h dialysis session. When water is drunk, protection against minor impurities, bacteria and toxins is afforded by the mucous membranes and acidity of the gastrointestinal tract; when a person is dialysed they are not protected in this way. It is therefore important that the quality of dialysis water is closely monitored.

Haemodialysis also involves the removal of excess fluid from the body. The process by which this is done is, by convention, called ultrafiltration. This process involves the dialysis machine putting less fluid into the dialyser than it removes. This creates a hydrostatic pressure across the dialysis membrane, called the transmembrane pressure, or TMP, and fluid (more or less just water) is removed from the blood (Terrill, 2002).

Haemodialysis requires that the blood is taken from the body, dialysed and returned to the body at a rapid rate. A good dialysis will involve passing all of the blood from the body through the dialyser several times. (During a 4-hour dialysis at a pump speed of 300 L a minute 72 L of blood is processed.) Access is the term used to describe the means by which blood is removed from, and returned to, the body and can be either a dialysis catheter, an arteriovenous fistula (see below), or a 'graft'.

Dialysis catheters are double-lumened tubes that are placed in major veins in the body; they are placed in the big veins in the neck, front of the shoulder or groin and can be temporary (used for a few weeks at most) or semipermanent (used for up to 2 or 3 years).

Opportunity for the student

Find out which veins are used to site dialysis catheters and why.
Most dialysis catheters are tunnelled under the skin. Find out why.

The preferred access for dialysis is the arteriovenous fistula. Fistulae are formed when an artery is surgically joined to a vein, causing the vein, which is not used to the pressures present in arteries, to swell. This swelling has a 'thrill' or 'bruit' when touched or listened to through a stethoscope because of the rapid, turbulent blood flow within it. Fistulae are preferred because they avoid the need for the insertion of a line, which is essentially a foreign body, and the incidence of infection is therefore greatly reduced (Terrill, 2002). Blood pressures should not be taken on an arm where fistulae have been formed to avoid damaging the fistula; neither should pulse oximetry be applied to a nearby finger as results will be erroneous due to the mixing of arterial and venous blood.

Opportunity for the student

What is the literal meaning of the word fistula?

Grafts are small tubes about 1 cm in diameter that are made from synthetic material (polytetrafluoroethylene or PTFE) similar to the non-stick material that is used in saucepans. Grafts are placed in individuals whose veins are not strong enough for a fistula to be created or in whom fistulae have failed. Grafts are placed between an artery and a vein and hence have a high blood flow, making them ideal for dialysis.

Large-bore needles are inserted into the fistula, or graft, to take blood away from and return blood to the patient during dialysis (Thomas, 2002). The positioning of these needles depends on the fistula, local policy and practice and the skill of the person, usually a nurse, placing them. Increasingly patients are being encouraged to self-care and may in fact place their own needles.

Reflection

The management of dialysis access is a specialist skill and it is advisable not to use them for anything other than dialysis except in an emergency situation. Why?

Most people dialyse for between 3 and 5 hours, two, or more normally three, times a week. The length of time that individuals dialyse depends on how much waste is in their blood. The amount of waste (creatinine and urea) that an individual produces depends on the amount of muscle that they have as well as the amount of protein in their diet. The length of time that individuals need to spend on dialysis is usually worked out by the dialysis staff who make calculations based on the amount of urea removed during each dialysis or on the size of the dialyser used and the approximate water content of the individual. Each patient has an individual dialysis prescription and the adequacy of dialysis is measured monthly.

Dialysis sessions using modern machines are associated with two main complications:

- Hypotension, or 'going flat': It occurs when water is being removed from the circulation quicker than it is being replaced from the interstitial space.
- Cramps: These can be quite severe and may occur when an individual is on the machine or at other times. Cramps also result from rapid water removal on dialysis, which reduces the flow of oxygenated blood to the muscles (Thomas, 2002).

Long-term complications of dialysis are related to the dialysis itself and also the underlying disease which caused the renal failure as well as other comorbidities. The most important complications include:

- Renal osteodystrophy, which is the result of altered calcium metabolism and is why many patients take calcium and vitamin D supplements
- Hypertension, which is often related to the increased fluid levels
- Heart disease, which occurs as a result of hypertension, anaemia, uraemic toxins and hypercholesterolaemia (usually high triglycerides)
- Pruritis (itching) from high phosphate levels

- Restless leg syndrome, which results from abnormal levels of electrolytes
- Fatigue, depression and psychological problems, also common and widely researched (Valderràbano et al., 2001)

The multidisciplinary team is important in the management of the psychological effects of life on dialysis. Communication skills, as discussed in Chapter 2, play an important role in the identification of patients with psychological problems. People on dialysis are more likely to develop depression than the general population. This has been attributed to the apparent hopelessness of life on dialysis, poor body image and physical symptoms (e.g. sleep disorders, poor appetite, weight loss, constipation and reduced libido) (Chiang et al., 2004).

Anger, which is quite common in patients on dialysis, sometimes shows itself as uncooperative behaviour, excessive drinking (water and other fluids) and non-adherence with prescribed medications. Sexual dysfunction is common among dialysis patients (Steggall and Gann, 2004) with up to 70% of men on dialysis being impotent, although sometimes the cause may be physical and not psychological.

The role of the dietician in enabling the patient to adapt their diet and fluid intake is integral to the work of the dialysis unit, while the pharmacist is important in advising and helping manage drug regimes. Social and occupational assessments are important in enabling dialysis patients to adjust to the everyday reality of being a dialysis patient.

Transplant clinic

The transplant clinic is often seen as the most exciting area of work in the renal department. The management of the patient both prior to and following kidney transplantation is itself a specialist job which employs the skills of all members of the inter-professional team.

Opportunity for the student

Find out what members of the inter-professional team are involved in the care and management of the patient who is working up for transplant?

Patients being prepared (worked up) for transplant may come from any of the other areas of the renal department. The most fortunate patients are those in the nephrology or low-clearance clinic who are being worked up for a pre-emptive live-related transplant and who will avoid the need for dialysis. Most patients will however come from the peritoneal dialysis or haemodialysis clinic.

There are three main sources of transplant kidneys:

- Cadaveric donors – people who have experienced brain death but whose hearts are beating and are on a ventilator
- Live donors – both genetically related (live-related) and emotionally related (live-unrelated) donors; often partners or spouses

- Non-heart-beating donors – involves using a machine which provides manual cardiac massage to individuals who have suffered sudden cardiac arrest as well as infusing a preserving solution into their kidney until permission to harvest the kidneys for transplantation is obtained from their next of kin.

Reflection

Some countries, like Spain, have an opt-out system for transplant donation. This means everyone is considered to be a potential donor unless, in life, they have expressly opted out. It has been argued that the UK should adopt such a system. What do you think are the ethical implications of such a scheme? Do you think it is a right or a wrong thing to do? Why?

The rules governing suitability for transplant are quite strict; this is to help maximise the success of the transplant itself and also to ensure that the transplant recipient themselves are likely to live for some years post-transplant.

In the pre-transplant clinic the patient who is being worked up for transplant is subjected to a number of tests and procedures to establish their suitability. The cause of the original renal disease needs to be taken into account first as many primary causes of renal disease will recur in the transplanted kidney causing it to become diseased. This means many patients with immunological causes for their renal failure may not be suitable transplant recipients. In many units infection with HIV, hepatitis B and C would prevent a patient from being considered for transplantation; other units deal with patients with these infections on an individual basis and with regard to the severity of their disease. Patients being worked up for transplant will have to be free from malignant disease, as the immunosuppression (antirejection drugs) used after surgery may cause the cancer to grow at a more rapid rate.

Patients with diabetes, as well as being likely to see a recurrence of the disease in their transplanted kidney, are also at increased risk of cardiovascular disease and careful consideration as to their suitability for transplant takes place before putting them on the transplant waiting list.

Human genes, which create the differences between individuals, will also cause transplants to be identified as foreign. Preparation for transplant therefore involves matching not only of blood group, but also of human leukocyte antigens particularly HLA-A, HLA-B and HLA-DR if these are not closely matched prior to transplantation. The recipient T cells will recognise the transplant as being foreign and attack it. Even the best-matched kidneys are in danger of being recognised as foreign and the patient will need life-long immunosuppression to protect the transplant kidney from being rejected. Some common immunosuppressive drugs and their side effects are included in Table 10.2.

These drugs work in different ways to block the immune responses. This means that they also make the body more prone to infections and cancers. There is a difficult balance to be achieved between preventing rejection and minimising side effects of immunosuppressive drugs and preventing rejection. Achieving this balance and managing the side effects employs the skills of many members of the

Table 10.2 Common immunosuppression drugs and their side effects

Drug	Side effects
Steroids	Gastric ulcer, hyperglycaemia, obesity, altered mood and poor wound healing
Azathioprine	Pancreatitis, bone marrow suppression causing neutropenia and thrombocytopenia
Mycophenolate	Gastric upset and diarrhoea
Cyclosporin and tacrolimus	Kidney damage, hirsutism, excessive gum growth, hyperkalaemia, hypertension
Sirolimus	Poor wound healing, neutropenia and thrombocytopenia

inter-professional team. Care is intensive in the first few months following transplant with gradually reducing visits to outpatients occurring over the following years and months.

Key roles of the inter-professional team in the transplant clinic include:

- Monitoring and controlling blood pressure (which may damage the transplant)
- Monitoring the urine for signs of infection
- Monitoring renal function via blood tests
- Controlling immunosuppression with reference to blood levels, kidney function, the presence and absence of side effects and white cell counts
- Monitoring for and treating infection vigorously
- Education about the occurrence of, and strategies to prevent/detect, early:
  - Anaemia
  - Infection
  - Weight gain
  - Skin cancer
  - Cardiovascular disease
  - Bone disease
  - Gum hyperplasia

Reflection

You could consider adding your name to the organ donor register at
http://www.uktransplant.org.uk/ukt/how_to_become_a_donor/how_to_become_a_donor.jsp

---

Many units now also have teams of staff that provide a service to those individuals who decide that they do not want to have dialysis, the conservative management team. This usually consists of a doctor, a nurse, a social worker/care manager, a counsellor/psychologist and a minister of religion. The role of this team is to provide ongoing symptom management and psychological support for patient often in their own homes. Members of this team liaise closely with staff in local hospices and general practice and share expertise regarding keeping conservatively managed patients as symptom free as is possible (Murtagh et al., 2006).

Scenario

Ms Drobkov, a 23-year-old Slovak with broken English, was referred from the MIU to the urology team for assessment following an acute episode of pyelonephritis (see Chapter 5). She has been referred on to the renal team for further assessment. The clinic nurse checks her blood pressure, her weight and dip-tests some urine.

(1) What is the significance of the observations?
(2) What might she/he find?

The nephrology consultant sees her after the clinic-based assessments and orders a series of further tests to determine the cause and extent of her problems. These tests include urea and electrolytes, full blood count, a urinary albumin-to-creatinine ratio and a renal ultrasound.

(1) Why are these tests undertaken?
(2) What might they show?

Summary

This chapter has identified the physiological functions of the kidneys, the causes, classifications and effects of renal disease; it has discussed some of the many outpatient settings in which renal care is provided and has acknowledged the important role that inter-professional working has in attaining a high quality of care. This chapter has not sought to fully explore the rich seam of knowledge, teamwork and care which renal units provide, but has gone some way towards demonstrating that renal outpatient areas provide a diverse, challenging and engaging place for the health student to gain a unique insight into true inter-professional, patient-centred care.

The author thanks Karen Jenkins, Nurse Consultant at the Kent and Canterbury Renal Unit, for commenting on this chapter.

Glossary of terms

Albumin
A common blood protein

Erythrocytes
Red blood cells

Erythropoiesis
Stimulating agents – drugs used to replace the hormone erythropoietin and stimulate the bone marrow to make red blood cells.

Erythropoietin
The hormone which stimulates red bone marrow to produce erythrocytes

Haematuria
Blood in the urine

Hypercholesterolaemia
High levels of cholesterol in the blood

Hypertrophy
Increase in size of a body organ or area of tissue

Hypoalbuminaemia
Low levels of albumin in the blood

Lumen
A channel

Nephropathy
Any disease of the kidneys

Occult
Hidden or not visible to the naked eye

Osteodystrophy
Any bone disorder

Proteinuria
Presence of protein, or albumin, in the urine

Protein-to-creatinine ratio
Used to measure protein in the urine

Retinopathy
Any disease process which affects the retina

SI units
These refer to the units of measurement agreed by both countries and therefore most commonly in use around the world. SI refers to the French système international d'unités

Stents
A tube inserted into a blood vessel, or other bodily passage, to keep the lumen open

Websites

http://renalworld.com/regions_links/index_html
http://patients.uptodate.com/toc.asp?toc=kidney_disease&title=Kidneydisease
http://www.renal.org/pages/
http://www.renalreg.com/

References

Chiang, C.K., Peng, Y.S., Chiang, S.S., Yang, C.S., He, Y.H., Hung, K.Y., Wu, K.D., Wu, M.S., Fang, C.C., Tsai, T.J. and Chen, W.Y. (2004) Health-related quality of life of hemodialysis patients in Taiwan: a multicenter study. *Blood Purification* 22(6), pp. 490–498.

Department of Health (DH) (2004) *The National Service Framework for Renal Services, Part One: Dialysis and Transplantation*. London: HMSO.

Department of Health (DH) (2005) *The National Service Framework for Renal Services, Part Two: Chronic Kidney Disease, Acute Renal Failure and End of Life Care*. London: HMSO.

Ellis, P.A. and Cairns, H.S. (2001) Renal impairment in elderly patients with hypertension and diabetes. *Quarterly Journal of Medicine 94*(5), pp. 261–265.

Ellis, P.A. (1997) Haemodialysis update. *Professional Nurse 13*(3), pp. 174–178.

Graham, C. (1998) Principles of peritoneal dialysis, in Challinor, P. and Sedgewick, J. (eds) *Principles and Practice of Renal Nursing*. Cheltenham: Stanley Thornes, pp. 167–183.

Jenkins, K. (2004) Anaemia management in nephrology, in Thomas, N. (ed.) *Advanced Renal Care*. Oxford: Blackwell Publishing, pp. 27–49.

Khan, I.H., Catto, G.R.D., Edward, N. and Macleod, A.M. (1994) Chronic renal failure: factors influencing nephrology referral. *Quarterly Journal of Medicine 87*(9), pp. 559–564.

Klang, B., Bjorvell, H. and Clyne, N. (1999) Predialysis education helps patients choose dialysis modality and increases disease-specific knowledge. *Journal of Advanced Nursing 29*, pp. 869–876.

Levy, J., Pusey, C. and Singh, A. (2006) Fast *Facts: Renal Disorders*. Oxford: Health Press.

Mahon, A. and Hattersley, J. (2002) Investigations in renal failure, in Thomas, N. (ed.) *Renal Nursing*, 2nd ed. London: Balliere Tindall, pp. 143–170.

Medline plus (2007) *Encyclopaedia: Duplex Ultrasound*. Available from: http://www.nlm.nih.gov/medlineplus/ency/article/003433.htm (accessed 12 July 2007).

Murtagh, F.E., Addington-Hall, J.M., Donohoe, P. and Higginson, I.J. (2006) Symptom management in patients with established renal failure managed without dialysis. *Journal of the European Dialysis and Transplant Nurses Association/European Renal Care Association 32*(2), pp. 93–98.

National Institute for Health and Clinical Excellence (NIHCE) (2006) *Anaemia Management in Chronic Kidney Disease: National Clinical Guideline in Adults and Children*. London: National Institute for Health and Clinical Excellence.

Sesso, R. and Yoshihiro, M.M. (1997) Time of diagnosis of chronic renal failure and assessment of quality of life in haemodialysis patients. *Nephrology Dialysis and Transplantation 12*, pp. 2111–2116.

Steggall, M. and Gann, S. (2004) Sexual dysfunction and renal disease, in Thomas, N. (ed.) *Advanced Renal Care*. Oxford: Blackwell Publishing, pp. 143–157.

Stein, A., Wild, J. and Cook, P. (2004) *Vital Nephrology*. London: Class Health.

Terrill, B. (2002) *Renal Nursing: A Guide to Practice*. Oxford: Radcliffe Medical Press.

Thomas, N. (2002) Haemodialysis, in Thomas, N. (ed.) *Renal Nursing*, 2nd ed. London: Balliere Tindall, pp. 171–206.

UK Renal registry (2006) *The Ninth Annual Report* [online]. Available from: http://www.renalreg.com/Report%202006/Cover_Frame2.htm (accessed 13 September 2007).

Valderràbano, F. Jofre, R. and Lopez-Gomez, J.M. (2001) Quality of life in end-stage renal disease patients. *American Journal of Kidney Diseases 38*, pp. 443–464.

Wild, J. (2002) Peritoneal dialysis, in Thomas, N. (ed.) *Renal Nursing*, 2nd ed. London: Balliere Tindall, pp. 207–266.

Further reading

Brook, N.R. and Nicholson, M.L. (2003) Clinical review: kidney transplantation from non heart-beating donors, *Journal of the Royal College of Surgeons of Edinburgh and Ireland 1*(6), pp. 311–322.

White, C.A., Pilkey, R.M., Lam, M. and Holland, D.C. (2002) Pre-dialysis clinic attendance improves quality of life among hemodialysis patients. *BMC Nephrology 3*(3) [online]. Available from: http://www.biomedcentral.com/1471-2369/3/3 (accessed 18 September 2007).

Chapter 11

Ambulatory cancer care

Paula Kuzbit

Learning objectives
By the end of this chapter you should be able to:

(1) Discuss ambulatory care in relation to cancer and the role of the nurse within this
(2) Describe how chemotherapy, radiotherapy and biotherapy work in the treatment of cancer
(3) Examine the supportive care needs of people with cancer within the ambulatory care setting

---

Introduction

Definition

Cancer care occurs in a wide variety of locations including inpatient facilities, primary care and the ambulatory care setting. Ambulatory cancer care refers to a care episode that lasts no longer than 23 hours and 59 min and which can be repeated over many days, months or even years (Buchsel and Henke Yarbro, 2005).

One in three people in the United Kingdom (UK) will develop cancer at some stage in their lifetime and it is responsible for over a quarter of all deaths in the UK; each year over 250 000 people are diagnosed and 150 000 die from the illness.

There are over 200 different types of cancer however; breast, lung, colorectal and prostate cancers make up half of all new cases (Cancer Research UK, 2005, 2006a). The population is ageing and, as a consequence, it is estimated that by the year 2025 an additional 100 000 people will be living with cancer (Cancer Research UK, 2006b). A considerable issue facing today's cancer services is the increasing number of treatment episodes required. Previously, patients may have received chemotherapy or radiotherapy only on one occasion. It is now common, however, for them to require both forms of treatment on multiple occasions. This has major implications when trying to ensure everyone receives equitable and timely treatment. New ways of working are therefore essential if cancer service providers are to meet this increasing demand.

It is estimated that approximately 80–90% of cancer care occurs within the ambulatory setting (Buchsel and Henke Yarbro, 2005; Downing, 2001). The move to ambulatory cancer care is being driven by three key factors: economic pressures, new technologies and changes within society itself. Escalating cancer care costs, new treatment strategies, changes in clinical practice and advances in managing the side effects of treatments are all placing pressure on already-stretched resources (Kearney and Richardson, 2006). Ambulatory cancer care provides specialist services to patients that are evidence based and user friendly. They have the capacity to expand and the ability to develop innovative approaches to care as the number of patients increase (Buchsel and Henke Yarbro, 2005).

This chapter will discuss ambulatory cancer care and the nurses' role within this service delivery model. It will go on to describe the principles that underpin the common cancer treatments and explore the supportive care needs of patients receiving these treatments.

Ambulatory cancer care

Innovations in treatments and the management of side effects now means many patients no longer have to stay in hospital; they can receive their care as an outpatient or day case, i.e. within ambulatory care. The concept of ambulatory care originated in the United States of America where health care costs were escalating and new ways of providing care were required to ensure sustainable services (Buchsel and Henke Yarbro, 2005). The United Kingdom, keen to develop twenty-first-century health care, has now adopted this innovative approach, where care is seen as a shared responsibility between the specialist cancer centre, the cancer unit, primary care and the patients themselves.

Services provided within ambulatory cancer care (ACC) are increasing rapidly and include screening, clinical investigations, day surgery, chemotherapy, biotherapy and radiotherapy treatments, as well as traditional new patient clinics, treatment review and follow-up clinics. Supportive cancer care is also provided as part of this growing service and may include blood component therapy, vascular access device insertion and maintenance, complementary therapy, pain and symptom management.

A person diagnosed with cancer begins a long and life-changing journey, where contact with cancer services often continues over many months or years.

Professional relationships need to be supportive, therapeutic and informative. Oncology departments have diverse and inclusive skill mixes, including registered nurses, health care support workers, therapy radiographers, dietitians, counsellors and oncologists, with each professional group having key areas of responsibility. Nurses, however, take a key role in the organisation of the patient's pathway (Grundy, 2006). Calman and Hine (1995) stated, in their national policy framework for cancer services, that patient care in both local units and specialist centres must be planned and led by nurses who possess a post-registration qualification in oncology.

The oncology nurse has a responsibility to ensure that the patient can access the support, advice and guidance they need at the appropriate time and to plan, implement and evaluate the care they receive. Downing (2001), in a study exploring the role of the nurse in oncology outpatients, suggested 11 key responsibilities within ambulatory care:

- Patient counselling
- Health care maintenance
- Primary care
- Patient education
- Therapeutic care
- Normative care
- Non-client-centred care
- Communication
- Documentation
- Planning
- Management
  (Downing, 2001, p. 53)

The most important roles for qualified nurses are communication and therapeutic care and, for those holding post-registration qualifications in cancer care, patient support, education and counselling. Nurses are moving away from the traditional 'handmaiden' role of assisting to one where their specialist skills and knowledge are integral to the whole patient experience (Downing, 2001). Nurses are developing new roles and responsibilities including patient information clinics and conducting treatment reviews and follow-up clinics.

The American Academy of Ambulatory Care Nurses (AAACN, 1997) identified 12 core characteristics of practice within ambulatory care, including nursing autonomy, patient advocacy, collaboration and client teaching. It is crucial that nurses develop competency within these to enable them to successfully care for patients (Martin and Xistris, 2005). Ambulatory care nurses have a brief window of time in which to build a therapeutic relationship that will allow them to do this; therefore, excellent communication skills are essential.

Reflection

Reflect on Chapter 2 on communication. What skills do you think you will need to support a patient receiving treatment for cancer within an ambulatory setting?

The role of the nurse within the ACC setting

As people receiving treatment for cancer move from the inpatient hospital setting to ambulatory services they will no longer have the security of health care professionals immediately at hand 24 hours a day. This requires patients to be fully informed about their illness and treatments, so they can participate fully in their care and recognise potentially life-threatening side effects before they become serious (Treacy and Mayer, 2000). It is the primary responsibility of doctors and nurses to provide patients with all the information they require to enable them to undertake this complex and possibly frightening task (Department of Health NHS Executive, 2000).

Information offers reassurance and instruction reduces anxiety and stress, improves the patient experience, increases concordance and results in self-care behaviours being adopted (Mills and Sullivan, 1999; Rutten et al., 2005; Van der Molen, 1999, 2000). Since the information needs of patients change with the health care setting, and with the increase in ambulatory care, patients need to be prepared to make decisions and deal with problems in the home (McCaughan and Thompson, 2000).

Information needs to be of the right sort and given at the right time. During the diagnosis and treatment phases patients want information regarding their disease, treatment options and treatment side effects (Rutten et al., 2005). Information should be provided in both written and verbal form (Oakley et al., 2000); it is well recognised that patients do not retain all the information they are given during consultations partly due to anxiety and shock. Printed information provides them with material that can be referred to at any time and shared with their family and other people of their choice.

Patients frequently state that they are dissatisfied with the quality of the information they receive or do not have sufficient amounts to enable them to actively participate in their care (Cardy et al., 2006; Cox et al., 2006; Mills and Sullivan, 1999); this may be in part due to health care professionals underestimating patients' desire for information or ability to understand medical language. Information must be provided at a rate that is comfortable for the patient as too much too quickly may overwhelm them (Van der Molen, 2000).

A study by James et al. (2007) looking at the information-seeking behaviour of cancer patients and their carers has highlighted the growing importance of the internet. They found that although few patients were accessing the internet directly, 48% of the 200 carers interviewed had accessed this resource and half of the 800 patient participants had used information from the internet that had been given to them by carers or friends. These findings have implications for nurses in ensuring that the information patients are reading comes from valid and reliable sources. James et al. (2007) conclude that the internet is an effective information resource and health-care-professional-directed access will broaden its role.

Macmillan Cancer Support, one of the UK's largest cancer charities, recently carried out a study that showed that a quarter of cancer patients felt abandoned by health and social care professionals when they were not in hospital (Cardy et al., 2006). Macmillan are urging the government to prioritise and fund services that will address the emotional, practical and information needs of people affected by cancer.

Within the ambulatory setting nurses are taking the lead in developing innovative services such as telephone triage. Telephone-based services offer a direct point of contact and access to instantaneous advice and guidance ranging from simple health promotion through to referral to specialist services and may reduce the feelings of abandonment experienced by patients. Further research is needed to ascertain the full impact of these new services.

Opportunity for the student

What online resources can you find that are available to patients who want to find out more information about their cancer and treatment?

Cancer treatments

Chemotherapy

There is evidence of the ancient Egyptians using substances, including arsenic, to treat conditions that may in today's society be classified as cancer. In its current form, however, chemotherapy has been an integral part of cancer treatments since the second half of the twentieth century. Historically, only used as palliative treatment, chemotherapy is now being more widely used with cure as the main goal and is one of the most important treatments in the fight against cancer (Brighton and Wood, 2005).

The term *chemotherapy* means the use of chemicals to destroy or kill cells, specifically malignant cells. The advantage of chemotherapy is that it can destroy cells throughout the body and is therefore a systemic treatment. However, chemotherapy does not only kill malignant cancer cells, but also kills healthy, non-cancerous ones. Chemotherapy destroys cells that are regularly undergoing the cell cycle; this not only includes cancer cells, but also includes skin, hair, mucosal and haemopoeitic cells (cells which are involved in the production of blood cells). It is because of this lack of ability to differentiate between healthy and cancerous cells that many of the common side effects of chemotherapy occur.

There have been many advances over the last 30 years that have changed the person with cancer's experience of chemotherapy, e.g. the increased availability of oral chemotherapy agents, improvements in side effect management and the development of home infusion devices. Now rather than patients having to stay in hospital whilst receiving treatment, they can be at home, living in their community surrounded by their support network.

Chemotherapy services are delivered in tertiary cancer centres, district general hospitals, primary care settings and the private health care sector. These developments bring with them a change in the focus of chemotherapy nursing from doing things for patients to empowering them to do things for themselves them. They also need to develop skills in patient education, information provision and psychosocial support to enable the patient to instigate self-care strategies essential for safe and effective treatment (Brighton and Wood, 2005; Coward and Coley, 2006; Department of Health, 2004).

Reflection

Reflect on how chemotherapy treatment is portrayed in the media. How might this affect the patients' understanding of the treatment?

How does chemotherapy work?

Cumulative knowledge

Before reading this section write down everything you know about chemotherapy. Once you have read this section review how your knowledge has progressed.

There are over 200 individual chemotherapy drugs each with different methods of causing cell death. However, they all primarily interact with the cell at varying points during the cell cycle.

Reflection

Review your knowledge of human anatomy and physiology relating to the normal cell cycle and cell division.

Each cell in the human body that replicates goes through a regulated, well-controlled process called the cell cycle (Figure 11.1). This five-phase process results in the production of an identical daughter cell (Marieb and Hoehn, 2007). G1 and G2 refer to gap phases where cellular growth occurs and the cell prepares for deoxyribonucleic acid (DNA) synthesis, or mitosis, to occur. There are a series of checkpoints within G1 and G2 which ensure that the cell is supported by a viable environment and that DNA has not sustained any damage and replication has occurred successfully. DNA replication occurs during the synthesis phase; here an exact copy of the original cellular DNA will be made. At mitosis the cell divides into two separate, but identical, cells. Lastly Gap 0 (zero) refers to those cells that are resting or not actively undergoing cell cycle. This may be permanent or cells can be recalled from G0 into cell cycle when the body requires replacements (Marieb and Hoehn, 2007).

Cancer is a disease of unregulated cell replication and growth, where many of the controls of the cell cycle and cell regulation are lost (Souhami and Tobias, 2005). Chemotherapy drugs interact with the cell at different stages within the cycle to cause irreparable damage and instigate cellular death; therefore, cells that are regularly going through this process will be most affected by chemotherapy.

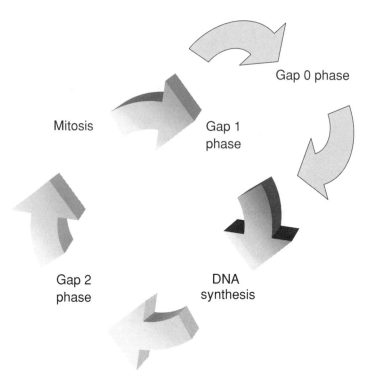

Figure 11.1   Cell cycle.

Chemotherapy can be divided into cell-cycle-specific and cell-cycle-non-specific drugs. Drugs which are cell cycle specific work at certain points within the cycle; for these to be effective the cell must be going through the cell cycle. For example, 5-fluorouracil replaces a vital component required to manufacture DNA bases during the synthesis phase. Drugs classified as non-specific do not rely on the cell being at a certain point to be able to exert a pharmacological action. This often means, however, that there will be greater toxic effects on normal health cells and therefore increased side effects (Coward and Coley, 2006) (Table 11.1).

Chemotherapy as treatment

Cancer is most sensitive to chemotherapy when there is a high percentage of cells going through the cell cycle. This is referred to as the growth fraction and tumour-doubling time. Tumours with a high growth fraction and a fast doubling time, e.g. testicular cancer, are sensitive to the effects of the drugs whereas tumours that are not as fast growing, e.g. colon cancer, are less sensitive. Chemotherapy is still very effective in the treatment of these cancers, but it may form one part of a multi-modal approach rather than being given on its own.

Chemotherapy is given in order to cure cancer, to extend life expectancy (where cure is not achievable) and to improve quality of life. In order to achieve these aims a variety of strategies are used:

Table 11.1 Classification of chemotherapy drugs.

Drug group	Mode of action	Cell cycle specific/ non-specific	Example drugs
Antimetabolites	Structural analogues of intracellular metabolites required for cell function and replication. Prevent DNA synthesis and result in cell death	S phase specific	5-Fluorouracil, methotrexate, cytarabine, gemcitabine, capecitabine
Antitumour antibiotics and anthracyclines	Act in numerous ways to inhibit DNA synthesis and replication	Non-specific	Daunorubicin, doxorubicin, epirubicin
Alkylating agents	Bind with DNA causing intra- and inter-strand cross linkages, resulting in DNA being unable to separate during replication	Non-specific	Cyclophosphamide, ifosfamide, chlorambucil, temozolomide, dacarbazine
Mitotic inhibitors	Inhibit the formation of mitotic spinals and bind to microtubules	G2/M phase specific	Docetaxel, paclitaxel, vincristine, vinorelbine,
Platinum agents	Interact with DNA causing cross linkages	Non-specific	Cisplatin, carboplatin, oxaliplatin
Topoisomerase inhibitors	Interact with topoisomerase I and II enzymes required for the accurate replication of DNA	Non-specific	Irinotecan, etoposide

Primary: Chemotherapy is the only treatment being used. Aim: curative.

Adjuvant: Chemotherapy is given after another form of cancer treatment, e.g. surgery or radiotherapy. Aim: curative.

Neoadjuvant: Chemotherapy is given prior to another form of treatment to 'down-stage' the tumour, so the second treatment is less invasive or more successful. Aim: curative.

Palliative: Chemotherapy is given to alleviate the symptoms the patient is experiencing and to increase life expectancy. Aim: not to cure the cancer.

Combination: More than one chemotherapy drug is given. Chemotherapy treatments are normally referred to as regimes, with the beginning letter of each drug making up the name of the regime. For example FEC consists of three drugs: 5-flurouracil, epirubicin and cyclophosphamide.

High-dose chemotherapy: Chemotherapy is given at very high doses in order to kill as many cancer cells as possible. This causes profound bone marrow suppression, leaving the patient with a very limited ability to fight infection or to stop bleeding. In order to help the patient recover they are given a peripheral blood stem cell transplant (PBSCT).

Modulation: A second drug is given with the chemotherapy drug to increase its effectiveness; e.g. folinic acid is often given with 5-flurouracil to increase its cell-killing actions.

Protective agents: A drug is given to the patient after the chemotherapy to help them recover from the effects of the treatment; e.g. folinic acid is given after methotrexate.

Chemotherapy is usually given in combinations of more than one drug and in treatment cycles. Each time chemotherapy is given, a constant percentage of cells is killed not a total number. Therefore repeated doses of chemotherapy are required to destroy the whole tumour (Skipper et al., 1964). Additionally in the time between treatments the tumour will continue to grow, chemotherapy therefore needs to be delivered at a point when healthy cells have had an opportunity to repair or be replaced but before the tumour can repopulate, this is referred to as a treatment cycle. The benefits of giving combinations of drugs include reduced resistance, less intense side effect profiles and killing cells at different points in the cell cycle, therefore maximising the effect of each chemotherapy cycle.

Administration of chemotherapy

Chemotherapy is administered via numerous routes, including:

- Intravenous
- Oral
- Intramuscular
- Intravesical (into the bladder)
- Intrapleural (into the pleural lining of the lung)
- Intraperitoneal (into the peritoneal cavity)
- Intrathecal (into the spinal canal)

Intravenous administration is the most common route. Patients may, for example, have a single intravenous injection, repeated weekly; a combination of short infusions and bolus injections given once every 3 weeks; or a continuous intravenous infusion via a central venous catheter and an ambulatory pump for up to 6 months (Figure 11.2).

There are a growing number of drugs that are given orally, e.g. capecitabine for colorectal cancer and vinorelbine for lung cancer. The increased use of oral chemotherapy drugs enables the patient to manage their treatment at home; however, as they are not visiting the hospital with the same frequency as other patients they might not have the same access to information, advice and support. Patients may feel unsupported or unsure about how to manage their own care. To avoid this, information on the toxicities they can expect and whom they should contact if they have any questions or concerns is vital. They also need access to ongoing support and guidance, whilst at home this is provided by both the primary health care team and the chemotherapy unit. An audit of oral chemotherapy telephone treatment reviews has shown that patients value being contacted by a nurse; they were able to

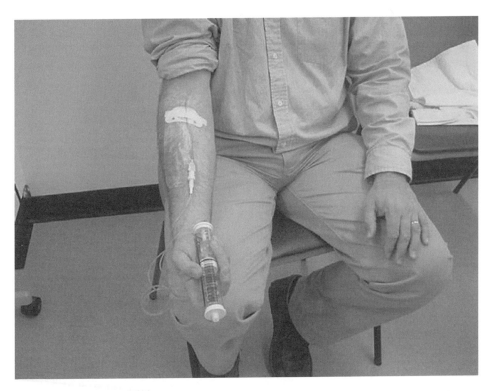

Figure 11.2 An ambulatory chemotherapy pump attached to a peripherally inserted central catheter (PICC).

acquire additional information, help and support with managing different aspects of their treatment (Lowe, 2007).

Side effects

The side effects of chemotherapy are varied; however, there are some common effects that patients experience (Table 11.2).

Bone marrow suppression is one of the most important and immediately life threatening side effects of chemotherapy. The white blood cells, called neutrophils, are the body's first defence against invading pathogens and replicate extraordinarily rapidly. As previously discussed chemotherapy attacks cells that undergo rapid replication; therefore, neutrophils are some of the most commonly affected cells in the body, having reduced numbers of neutrophils called neutropenia. This effect normally occurs within 7 to 14 days of each treatment cycle. Neutropenic patients are at much greater risk of developing infections, potentially leading to sepsis. Therefore it is essential that patients and health care professionals are alert to the early signs of infection so that antibiotics can be given quickly.

Patients should be advised to contact their local chemotherapy unit if they develop a raised temperature or flulike symptoms, as they may not be aware they are neutropenic and these may be the first signs of infection. A patient suspected of

Table 11.2 Common side effects and example chemotherapy drugs

Nausea and vomiting	High risk: • Cisplatin • Carboplatin • Doxorubicin • Epirubicin • Oxaliplatin • Lomustine Moderate risk: • Etoposide • Doxetaxel • Paclitaxel • Cytarabine • Methotrexate (high dose) Low risk: • 5-Fluorouracil • Bleomycin • Methotrexate (low dose) • Chlorambucil • Vinca alkaloids
Bone marrow suppression (reduced white cell and platelet production)	Most chemotherapy drugs will cause bone marrow suppression to varying degrees, examples include: • Doxorubicin • Methotrexate • Carboplatin • Cytarabine • Irinotecan
Alopecia (hair loss)	Not all chemotherapies cause alopecia, examples of drugs that do include: • Epirubicin • Doxorubicin • Cyclophosphamide • Etoposide • Paclitaxel
Fatigue	All chemotherapy appears to cause a degree of fatigue due to a number of factors. The pattern of fatigue depends on the regime the patient is having and how it is delivered
Change in bowel habits	Diarrhoea: • 5-Fluorouracil • Capecitabine • Irinotecan • Cisplatin (high dose) • Cytarabine • Docetaxel • Paclitaxel • Mitomycin Constipation: • Oxaliplatin • Vincristine • Vinorelbine

being neutropenic should be treated as an emergency. Observations must be taken, and samples, including full blood count, wound swabs and blood cultures, will be required to ascertain whether they are neutropenic; if they have an infection, then to identify the invading pathogen. The neutropenic patient should be regularly monitored as their condition can change very rapidly; this monitoring includes regular temperature, pulse, respiration and blood pressure recordings, increasing in frequency if any findings are abnormal.

Nausea and vomiting are common side effects and may be debilitating for the patient. Supportive care should be instigated immediately to avoid the patient developing any complications. Commonly used antiemetics include the 5-HT$_3$ antagonists, ondansetron and granisetron administered by tablet or intravenous injection for immediate or severe nausea and vomiting and the dopamine antagonists metaclopramide and domperidone for ongoing or moderate symptoms. The corticosteroid dexamethasone is also given as part of the regime; however, its mode of action is not fully understood. Patients should be sent home with a supply of the appropriate antiemetic and advised to contact the chemotherapy unit if they experience any breakthrough nausea or vomiting.

It is a common misconception amongst the public that all chemotherapies cause hair loss. This is not the case. Chemotherapy drugs can cause complete alopecia, partial alopecia or do not affect the hair at all. Hair loss is transitory and hair will grow back within weeks of completing treatment. The impact of hair loss can be distressing and may lead to devastating changes to body image perception, loss of self-esteem and confidence (Batchelor, 2006; Kuzbit, 2004). Nurses, therefore, need to help prepare the patient for the impact of alopecia and discuss the benefits of interventions including scalp cooling (Kuzbit, 2004).

Radiotherapy

Radiotherapy has been part of the cancer treatment armoury for approximately 100 years. It is the second most effective form of treatment after surgery; 50% of patients will require it during their cancer journey and 60% of these receive it with the intention of curing the disease (Burnet et al., 2000). Radiotherapy is delivered mostly as an outpatient in specially designed treatment centres. Nursing is focused on education, assessment and the psychosocial needs of the patient and their family (Blay et al., 2002). As with many cancer treatments there are numerous myths and inaccuracies that have developed leading to increased fear and anxiety for the patient. One of the key roles of the health care team is to reduce this level of anxiety and allay any fears regarding the treatment process.

How does radiotherapy work?

Radiotherapy uses high-energy X-rays to produce ionising radiation that obliterate cells within a treatment area. It will destroy both cancerous and healthy cells. The main target of the radiation beam is cellular DNA. Radiation will cause a break in one, or both, of the strands of the DNA double helix, resulting in either immediate cellular death or death during replication (Faithfull, 2006). Cells that undergo frequent replication are most affected by radiotherapy (Watson et al., 2006). Unlike systemic treatments, the effects of radiotherapy are largely confined to the area being treated; it is therefore considered a local treatment. The side effects that the patient experiences are related to the area; e.g. diarrhoea may occur when the bowel is being irradiated.

There are differences in the ways that tumours respond to radiation; this is referred to as radiosensitivity; some cancers are more sensitive to irradiation than others. Factors that influence this include:

- Oxygenation: A tumour with a good oxygen supply will be more sensitive to radiation.
- The number of cancer cells actively dividing: The higher the proportion of cells replicating within the tumour the more sensitive it will be.
- The rate at which the tumour repopulates: When cancer cells have been destroyed, the tumour will attempt to replace those killed. It is therefore essential that patients do not miss or delay treatments (Burnet et al., 2000).
- Cellular repair: Cells can repair the damage caused by radiation; however, malignant cells are less able to do this than normal cells, allowing tissues to recover from the treatment.

How is radiotherapy given?

Radiotherapy is given for three key reasons:

- *Radical treatment*; curative intent. Radiotherapy is the primary treatment, often used when a patient does not want, or would not cope with, surgery.
- *Adjuvant treatment*; curative intent. Once the tumour has been removed surgically radiotherapy is used to treat any residual microscopic disease.
- *Palliative treatment*; radiotherapy is used to control symptoms when the cancer is not curable.

Cumulative knowledge

Before reading the next section revisit Chapter 7 to refresh your knowledge of radiological imaging techniques.

Before radiotherapy can begin patients have to attend a series of preparatory appointments to plan their individual treatment. X-rays, CT or MRI scans are taken to identify the tumour site, volume and shape. These scans are entered into computer programmes for a detailed map to be drawn, identifying exactly where the radiation beams need to be directed avoiding any vital organs adjacent to, or behind, the tumour. The treatment area will be marked on the patient's skin using tattoo ink; this allows the therapy radiographer to ensure that the right area is treated each time; however, patients may feel branded or stigmatised by these (Wells, 2003a). Patients receiving radiotherapy to the head and neck, or brain, require an immobilisation shell. This shell is used to ensure the patient does not move during

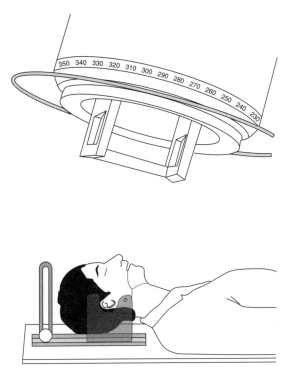

Figure 11.3   Head position for radiotherapy. The illustration shows how the head is held still using a clear mould so that external radiotherapy can be given. [Reproduced with permission, © Clinical Skills Ltd.]

the radiotherapy and the correct area is treated each time. However, having to use an immobilisation device can be a frightening and distressing experience especially for patients with claustrophobia or breathing difficulties (Wells, 2003a). Once all the plans are complete and any immobilisation device made the patient can commence treatment.

Treatment is usually given as external beam therapy called teletherapy (Figure 11.3). The high-energy X-ray is produced by a machine called a linear accelerator (linac). Patients lay under the linac on a hard couch, as they would if they were having an ordinary X-ray. They do not feel any pain from the actual radiation whilst it is being delivered; however, the position they have to lie in or the hardness of the couch may cause discomfort. The energy beam is aimed at the tumour site with the dose of radiation being calculated to enable the radiation to penetrate to a specific depth into the tissues. The actual treatment lasts only a few minutes; however, getting into the right position to receive this may take several more.

The unit of measure for dose of radiation is the Gray (Gy).

1 gray = 1 joule/kg

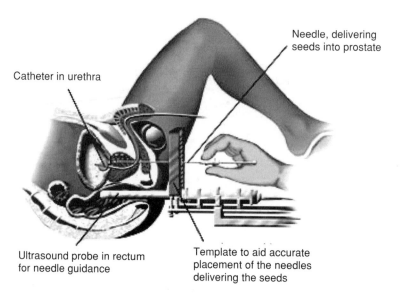

Catheter in urethra

Needle, delivering
seeds into prostate

Ultrasound probe in rectum
for needle guidance

Template to aid accurate
placement of the needles
delivering the seeds

Figure 11.4 Prostate brachytherapy. The picture shows how in prostate brachytherapy the sealed radiation source is placed inside the prostate gland. [Reproduced with permission, © Prostate Cancer Centre.]

Radiotherapy is given over a period of weeks, normally Monday to Friday. Patients are prescribed a dose of radiation that is known to have maximum effect on their type of cancer. This is then equally divided into small daily treatments: e.g. a patient may be prescribed 55 Gy over 5 weeks; this means they will receive 2.2 Gy/day (i.e. 2.2 Gy for 5 days a week). This division of the treatment allows for a high total dose to be given but enables healthy cells to repair in between treatments and is referred to as fractionation (Adamson, 2003).

Radiotherapy can also be given internally; this is called brachytherapy. A sealed radioactive source is placed next to the tumour, directly delivering the radiation dose. The main benefit of this treatment is surrounding healthy tissues are exposed to minimal amounts of radiation, therefore reducing the side effects. This type of therapy can be used for, among others, cervical and prostate cancers (Figure 11.4). A third type of radiotherapy is the use of radioisotopes, e.g. iodine (I^{131}) a systemic oral treatment used for thyroid cancer.

Common side effects associated with radiotherapy

All patients receiving radical radiotherapy will experience acute side effects which are often debilitating and impact on quality of life (Colyer, 2003; Faithfull, 2006). The majority are directly related to the area that is being treated. Fatigue, however, is a general side effect that affects most patients receiving radiotherapy (Kuzbit, 2002). Radiotherapy side effects develop and worsen over the period of the treatment and often continue for weeks or months after it has finished and a small proportion of patients may develop late side effects occurring 6 months to 2 years after the treatment has finished (Colyer, 2003; Table 11.3).

Table 11.3 Common side effects of radiotherapy and site treated

Side effects	Site treated
Xerostomia (dry mouth)	Mouth
Radiation skin reactions	Any area especially skinfolds
Mucositis (inflammation and ulceration of the mucus membranes)	Head and neck
Eosophagitis and dysphagia	Head and neck and oesophagus
Nausea and vomiting	Upper gastrointestinal tract
Diarrhoea	Lower gastrointestinal tract
Tenesmus (feeling of incomplete bowel evacuation and pain), cystitis and urethritis	Pelvic area

---

Opportunity for the student

Apart from fatigue what other general effects of radiotherapy might a patient experience?

One of the most common local side effects is radiation-induced skin damage. This occurs as a consequence of suppressed cellular replication and inflammatory reactions (Naylor, 2004). Mild skin reactions occur in approximately 80–90% of patients with severe moist desquamation occurring in 10–15% (Faithfull, 2006). Patients should be provided with in-depth information on caring for their skin (see Table 11.4).

When skin breaks down (moist desquamation) moist wound healing principles should be adopted. The use of hydrocolloids, hydrogels and alginates are all recommended; however, there is a lack of evidence regarding the best dressings to use (Faithfull, 2006; Naylor, 2004). Where available local policies should be referred to. Pain associated with radiotherapy skin reactions can be severe; patients should be frequently assessed and appropriate analgesia (including opiates) commenced.

Mucositis will occur when a patient is having treatment to the head and neck. Patients may also experience dry mouth (due to the destruction of salivary glands), eating difficulties, taste changes and pain. These may become so severe that patients

Table 11.4 Advice to patients on skin care

Gentle washing with mild unperfumed soap

Pat dry; do not rub

Avoid shaving or use an electric razor

Avoid perfumed products and deodorants

Wear loose, cotton clothing

Protect the area from wind, sun and extremes of temperature

Use simple moisturisers on unbroken areas

Faithfull, 2006; The College of Radiographers, 2001; Wells and MacBride, 2003.

require the insertion of a percutaneous endoscopic gastrostomy tube (PEG) for feeding. Excellent mouth care is essential to avoid infection; however, the usefulness of mouthwashes is controversial (Wells, 2003b). Normal saline rinses and optimum pain control provide the cornerstone of supportive care for patients with mucositis. Topical analgesia may be beneficial in the early stages including aspirin and paracetamol gargles, and agents such as artificial saliva replacements may be helpful (Watson et al., 2006).

Patients experiencing diarrhoea should be advised to reduce their dietary roughage and may require antidiarrhoeal agents. Nausea and vomiting should be controlled with antiemetic therapy (Watson et al., 2006).

Opportunity for students

What advice should a woman receiving radiotherapy to the breast receive regarding skin care?

Radiotherapy is often seen as routine and not as debilitating as chemotherapy; however, in reality, it is very emotionally and physically demanding. The daily trips to hospital, often many miles away, and attempting to carry on day-to-day living around the treatment can often lead to exhaustion and anxiety. Patients require high levels of supportive care throughout their treatment and nurses, in collaboration with their radiotherapy and medical colleagues, are in a perfect position to offer this support. Patients are assessed daily by the therapy radiographer. The impact of the treatment can be reviewed and advice, or prompt side effect management, can be instigated, e.g. wound dressings, nutritional support or pain management. Interprofessional teams provide these and many other interventions where traditional roles and responsibilities are often abandoned in favour of holistic, patient-centred care.

Biotherapy

Biotherapy is the newest weapon in the cancer treatment armoury. It is an exciting time for the fourth treatment modality; discoveries into cancer biology and innovations in treatment are being made every day and patients are seeing the benefits of these discoveries directly. Biotherapy is defined as the use of naturally occurring biological molecules, including antibodies and cytokines, to target cancer cells in order to inhibit, control or destroy the tumour (Kerr et al., 2006; Table 11.5).

Biological therapies have varied ways of working; however, the basic principles behind them include binding with cancer cells and blocking signalling pathways, as with monoclonal antibodies, blocking the production of molecules that may encourage the cancer to grow, e.g. oestrogen, or promoting the replacement of cells that have been destroyed by other treatments, e.g. granulocyte colony-stimulating factor.

Biotherapies have very diverse and potentially severe side effects; nurses administering these need to be fully conversant with how to manage any adverse event that may occur during the therapy and also provide information and support to the patient at home. Common side effects include chills and rigors, fever, body

Table 11.5 Current biotherapy strategies and example agents

Hormonal therapy	Tamoxifen Anastrozole (Arimidex) Goserelin (Zoladex) Megestrol acetate (Megace)
Cytokine therapy	Interferon Interleukin
Haemopoietic growth factors	Granulocyte colony-stimulating factor Granulocyte-macrophage colony-stimulating factor Erythropoietin
Monoclonal antibodies	Trastuzumab (Herceptin) Rituximab Alemtuzumab
Others	Gene therapy Cancer vaccines Antiangiogenic drugs

pains, fatigue, allergic reactions and skin reactions. Management of these depends on the specific therapy and other concurrent treatments; following local guidelines is therefore essential.

Scenario

Mrs Green, 42, is referred to the oncology ambulatory clinic following excision of the impalpable breast lump. Unfortunately, investigations indicated an active form of tumour and subsequent lymph node sampling suggested tumour cell migration requiring further treatment.

(1) Describe the process by which cells migrate from the primary tumour to distant sites.
(2) What are the information needs of patients receiving chemotherapy?
(3) What would be the expected side effects of chemotherapy treatment and how might these be managed?

Summary

This chapter has explored ambulatory cancer care and how this new way of delivering services is developing within the UK. The nurse's role is fundamental in supporting patients. It is essential that they provide in-depth information and education to ensure the safety of the patient whilst they are at home. High levels of psychosocial and physical support are of paramount importance. The role of chemotherapy, radiotherapy and biotherapy in the treatment of cancer has been described with implications for nursing practice being highlighted. The three treatment modalities are very different in their mode of actions; however, there are many similarities in the physical and emotional toll that is placed on the patient and their families. Supporting patients through this journey is highly complex but rewarding work.

Glossary of terms

Ambulatory cancer care
Ambulatory cancer care refers to a care episode that lasts no longer than 23 hours and 59 minutes and can be repeated over many days, months or even years

Biotherapy
The use of naturally occurring biological molecules to target cancer cells in order to inhibit, control or destroy the tumour

Brachytherapy
Internal radiation

Cancer
Unregulated cell replication and growth, where many of the controls of the cell cycle and cell regulation are lost, resulting in the formation of a mass, local invasion and spread to other sites within the body

Cell cycle
The process by which cells replicate to produce an identical daughter cell

Chemotherapy
The use of drugs that kill cells to treat cancer

Curative
Treatment that is aimed at curing cancer

Neutropenia
Reduction in the number of neutrophils in the blood

Moist desquamation
Breakdown of the skin at the site of radiotherapy. Treatment symptoms include sloughing, blistering and weeping of serous fluid

Palliative
Treatment that is aimed at prolonging life expectancy, reducing symptoms and improving quality of life

Radiotherapy
The use of ionising radiation to treat cancer

Scalp cooling
The use of frozen gel caps or mains-powered cooling systems to lower the temperature of the scalp in order to restrict blood flow to the hair follicle and prevent alopecia

Teletherapy
External beam radiotherapy

Tumour doubling time
The time it takes for a tumour mass to double in size

Websites

Cancer Backup
http://www.cancerbackup.org.uk/Home
Cancer Help
http://www.cancerhelp.org.uk/
Cancer Research UK
http://www.cancerresearchuk.org/
Department of Health: Cancer
http://www.dh.gov.uk/en/Policyandguidance/Healthandsocialcaretopics/
Cancer/index.htm
Macmillan Cancer Support
http://www.macmillan.org.uk/Home.aspx
National Cancer Institute
http://www.cancer.gov/

References

Adamson, D. (2003) The radiobiological basis of radiation side effects, in Faithfull, S. and Wells, M. (eds.) *Supportive Care in Radiotherapy*. Edinburgh: Churchill Livingstone.

American Academy of Ambulatory Care Nursing (1997) *Nursing in Ambulatory Care: The Future is Here*. Washington, DC: American Nurses Publishing.

Batchelor, D. (2006) Alopecia, in Kearney, N. and Richardson, A. (eds) *Nursing Patients with Cancer Principles and Practice*. Edinburgh: Elsevier Churchill Livingstone.

Blay, N., Cairns, J., Chisholm, J. and O'Baugh, J. (2002) Research into the workload and roles of oncology nurses working within an outpatient oncology unit. *European Journal of Oncology Nursing* 6(1), pp. 6–12.

Brighton, D. and Wood, M. (2005) *Royal Marsden Hospital Handbook of Cancer Chemotherapy*. Edinburgh: Elsevier Churchill Livingstone.

Buchsel, P. and Henke Yarbro, C. (2005) *Oncology Nursing in the Ambulatory Setting*, 2nd ed. Boston: Jones and Bartlett.

Burnet, N., Benson, R., Williams, M. and Peacock, J. (2000) Improving outcomes through radiotherapy. *British Medical Journal 320*, pp. 198–199.

Calman, K. and Hine, D. (1995) *A Policy Framework for Commissioning Cancer Services: A Report by the Expert Advisory Group on Cancer to the Chief Medical Officers of England and Wales*. London: Department of Health.

Cancer Research UK (2005) *CancerStats Mortality UK*. Available from: http://info.cancerresearchuk.org/images/pdfs/cs_mortality_sept_2005.pdf (accessed 7 September 2007).

Cancer Research UK (2006a) *CancerStats Incidence – UK*. Available from: http://info.cancerresearchuk.org/images/pdfs/cs_incidence_feb_2006.pdf (accessed 7 September 2007).

Cancer Research UK (2006b) *Statistics on the Risk of Developing Cancer*. Available from: http://info.cancerresearchuk.org/cancerstats/incidence/risk/ (accessed 21 June 2007).

Cardy, P., Corner, J., Evans, J., Jackson, N., Shearn, K. and Sparham, L. (2006) *Worried Sick: The Emotional Impact of Cancer*. London: Macmillan Cancer Support.

Colyer, H. (2003) The context of radiotherapy care, in Faithfull, S. and Wells, M. (eds) *Supportive Care in Radiotherapy*. Edinburgh: Churchill Livingstone.

Cox, A., Jenkins, V., Catt, S., Langridge, C. and Fallowfield, L. (2006) Information needs and experiences: an audit of UK cancer patients. *European Journal of Oncology Nursing* 10, pp. 263–272.

Coward, M. and Coley, H. (2006) Chemotherapy, in Kearney, N. and Richardson, A. (eds) *Nursing Patients with Cancer Principles and Practice*. Edinburgh: Elsevier Churchill Livingstone.

Department of Health (DH) (2004) *Manual for Cancer Services*. Available from: http://www.dh.gov.uk/en/Publicationsandstatistics/Publications/PublicationsPolicyAnd Guidance/DH_4090081 (accessed 5 September 2007).

Department of Health NHS Executive (2000) *Cancer Information Strategy* Available from: http://www.dh.gov.uk/en/Publicationsandstatistics/Publications/PublicationsPolicyAnd Guidance/DH_4005424 (accessed 21 July 2007).

Downing, J. (2001) Oncology out-patients nursing: a challenge within the changing face of cancer care. *European Journal of Oncology Nursing* 5(1), pp. 49–59.

Faithfull, S. (2006) Radiotherapy, in Kearney, N. and Richardson, A. (eds) *Nursing Patients with Cancer Principles and Practice*. Edinburgh: Elsevier Churchill Livingstone.

Grundy, M. (2006) Cancer care and cancer nursing, in Kearney, N. and Richardson, A. (eds) *Nursing Patients with Cancer Principles and Practice*. Edinburgh: Elsevier Churchill Livingstone.

James, N., Daniels, H., Rahman, R., McConkey, C., Derry, J. and Young, A. (2007) A study of information seeking by cancer patients and their carers. *Clinical Oncology 19*, pp. 356–362.

Kearney, N. and Richardson, A. (2006) *Nursing Patients with Cancer Principles and Practice*. Edinburgh: Elsevier Churchill Livingstone.

Kerr, D., Rowett, L. and Young, A. (2006) *Cancer Biotherapy: An Introductory Guide*. Oxford: Oxford University Press.

Kuzbit, P. (2002) Improving the patient's experience of cancer related fatigue. *Cancer Nursing Practice 1*(9), pp. 31–37.

Kuzbit, P. (2004) The importance of hair. *Cancer Nursing Practice 3*(8), pp. 10–13.

Lowe, S. (2007) *An Audit of Patient Satisfaction of Nurse-Led Oral Chemotherapy Clinic: Pilot Study*. Unpublished

Marieb, E. and Hoehn, K. (2007) *Human Anatomy and Physiology*, 7th ed. San Francisco: Pearson Benjamin Cummings.

Martin, V. and Xistris, D. (2005) Ambulatory care, in Henke-Yarbro, C., Hansen Frogge, M. and Goodman, M. (eds) *Cancer Nursing Principles and Practice*, 6th ed. Boston: Jones and Bartlett Publishers.

McCaughan, E. and Thompson, K. (2000) Information needs of cancer patients receiving chemotherapy at a day case unit in Northern Ireland. *Journal of Clinical Nursing 9*(6), pp. 851–858.

Mills, M. and Sullivan, K. (1999) The importance of information giving to patients newly diagnosed with cancer: a review of the literature. *Journal of Clinical Nursing 8*(6), pp. 631–642.

Naylor, W. (2004) Wound management, in Dougherty, L. and Lister, S. (eds) *Royal Marsden Manual of Clinical Nursing Procedures*, 6th ed. Oxford: Blackwell Publishing.

Oakley, C., Wright, E. and Ream, E. (2000) The experiences of patients and nurses with a nurse led peripherally inserted central venous catheter line service. *European Journal of Oncology Nursing 4*(4), pp. 207–218.

Rutten, L., Arora, N., Bakos, A., Aziz, N. and Rowland, J. (2005) Information needs and sources of information among cancer patients: a systematic review of research (1980–2003). *Patient Education and Counselling 57*, pp. 250–261.

Skipper, H., Schabel, F. and Wilcox, W. (1964) Experimental evaluation of potential anti-cancer agents: XII. On the criteria and kinetics associated with the curability of experimental leukaemia. *Cancer Chemotherapy Reports 35*, pp. 1–11.

Souhami, R. and Tobias, J. (2005) *Cancer and Its Management*, 5th ed. Oxford: Blackwell Publishing.

The College of Radiographers (2001) *Summary of Intervention for Acute Radiotherapy Induced Skin Reactions in Cancer Patients.* London: RCR.

Treacy, J. and Mayer, D. (2000) Perspectives on cancer patient education. *Seminars in Oncology Nursing 16*(1), pp. 47–56.

Van Der Molen, B. (1999) Relating information needs to the cancer experience: 1 Information as a key coping strategy. *European Journal of Cancer Care 8*(4), pp. 238–244.

Van Der Molen, B. (2000) Relating information needs to the cancer experience. 2 themes from six cancer narratives. *European Journal of Cancer Care 9*(1), pp. 48–54.

Watson, M., Barrett, A., Spense, R. and Twelves, C. (2006) *Oncology*, 2nd ed. Oxford: Oxford University Press.

Wells, M. (2003a) The treatment trajectory, in Faithfull, S. and Wells, M. (eds) *Supportive Care in Radiotherapy.* Edinburgh: Churchill Livingstone.

Wells, M. (2003b) Oropharyngeal effects of radiotherapy, in Faithfull, S. and Wells, M. (eds) *Supportive Care in Radiotherapy.* Edinburgh: Churchill Livingstone.

Wells, M. and MacBride, S. (2003) Radiation skin reactions, in Faithfull, S. and Wells, M. (eds) *Supportive Care in Radiotherapy.* Edinburgh: Churchill Livingstone.

Chapter 12

Day hospital nursing

Colin Wheeldon

Learning objectives

After reading the chapter the reader will be able to:

(1) Define the role of the day hospital
(2) Identify key nursing opportunities
(3) Define health promotion activities in this care setting
(4) Identify potential nursing role developments

Introduction

Definition

The day hospital supports patients that need up to 8 hours of care during the daytime. It provides consultation, diagnostic function tests and defined time-limited multidisciplinary rehabilitation care packages of 6–12 weeks for predominantly older people.

In its National Service framework (NSF) for older people (Department of Health (DH), 2001) the UK government set out to ensure that older people were supported by integrated services with well coordinated, coherent and cohesive approaches to assessing patients' needs and circumstances. This was envisaged to increase access and reduce the cost burden of ill health on services and individuals in the older age bracket (DH, 2003). The focus is on promoting better health and increasing participation through socialisation activities to reduce the sense of isolation and psychological deterioration that can occur as older people are left on their own (DH, 2004). Provision specifically addresses those conditions which are particularly significant for older people, such as strokes, falls, respiratory and mental health problems associated with ageing. Health care professionals promote the health and well-being of older people through coordinated actions in health teams which aim to maintain patient independence and prevent unnecessary hospital or long-term residential care admission. The multidisciplinary approach includes outpatient assessment, treatment and rehabilitation (Dasgupta et al., 2005). Referrals are received from hospital and primary care for patients who have suffered strokes, falls or who have neurological disorders (e.g. Parkinson's disease), respiratory disease and/or mobility problems. Increasingly, day hospitals are also being used for other work such as blood transfusions, intravenous therapies, venesection and procedural aftercare such as that required after liver biopsies.

This chapter explores the context of care and range of services available and then moves forward to consider how roles and teamworking are implemented. In particular, it examines the nursing contribution to day hospital care and opportunities for nursing to become more defined in this setting. Health promotion and communication are considered in relation to specific patient groups that attend the day hospital. The chapter concludes by considering a shift in emphasis to adult medical ambulatory care and the opportunities for development that this provides.

Context of care

The first day hospital was opened in the UK in 1952 (Farndale, 1961) and developed rapidly in the 1960s as part of wider changes in the health care provision for older people designed to complement the care provided by inpatient services. The main purpose could be seen as prolonging independent living through specialist assessment and treatment of older people enabling them to remain in their own homes. The past 50 years have seen many changes in the type of services provided by day hospitals. A range of services such as specialist clinics for patients with falls, Parkinson's disease, heart failure, transient ischaemic episodes, as well as rapid access clinics have been added to the traditional multi-professional rehabilitation model for older people. The model has since been widely applied in New Zealand, Australia, Canada, the USA and several European countries (Forster et al., 2006).

Day hospital care offers more effective rehabilitation than no intervention at all, but may have little advantage over other forms of comprehensive elderly services. Although day hospitals appear expensive, their benefits include reduced inpatient bed use, avoiding hotel costs and utilising less institutional care by enabling the patient to retain more independence and stay in their own homes with health care support

(Potter and Perry, 2001), suggesting the potential for long-term cost-effectiveness (Forster et al., 2006). Savings, however, may be masked by becoming spread over a number of different budgets and multidisciplinary codes and therefore go unnoticed. Many such savings have also been consumed by bed-blocking issues so prevalent in the last decade.

Critics of comparisons between inpatient and day patient treatment emphasise that like is not being compared with like (Hildick-Smith, 1984, cited in Hershkovitz et al., 2003, p. 750). Day hospital treatment relates more closely to independence and accords with the wishes of most patients and families to receive their care whilst living at home. Costing involves not only money, but staffing, and here the day hospital continues to show advantage. Not only do day hospitals attract nurses and therapists, but a nurse can maintain ten times as many patients in the day hospital as he/she can in the wards. Over 80% of day hospital patients have help at home from a chief carer (family member, neighbour, friend or home help), and these helpers greatly increase the number available to care for the older person at home. This is a vital factor in the comparison of costs between day hospital and inpatient care (Hildick-Smith, 1984, cited in Hershkovitz et al., 2003, p. 750).

The initial aim of day hospitals was to ease the discharge process for older people, through continued supervision and monitoring, following a period of hospitalisation (Cosin, 1954, cited in Booth and Waters, 1995, p. 701). Over the past four decades the focus of day hospitals has changed in favour of active treatment and rehabilitation to maintain independence, and it is now generally accepted that day hospitals provide multidisciplinary assessment and rehabilitation facilities. The day hospital often provides the only social contact that patients may have as well as ensures vital respite for their carers. This respite facility allows family members to maintain their lifestyles and employment whilst still being able to care for their relatives in their own homes (Luekenotte, 2000). This mixed economy of care provision for older patients means that they can avoid admission to long-term full-time care facilities such as nursing or residential homes.

Day hospitals usually operate on a 5-day-a-week basis opening during business hours. They are often associated with, and managed by, NHS hospital trusts, although some are located in primary care facilities. The types of services provided by day hospitals include transportation to and from the day hospital, assistance with personal hygiene, nursing and therapeutic services (including counselling and rehabilitation), meals and recreational activities (Luekenotte, 2000).

Implementation of nursing and team roles

Nurses provide continuation of care between that delivered at home and in the day hospital (Potter and Perry, 2001). For example, ensuring the patient continues to take their prescribed medication. Ebersole and Hees (1998, cited in Potter and Perry, 2001, p. 35) suggest that knowledge of community needs and resources is essential in providing adequate support for patients who often spend only a few hours a week in the day care setting. The team members who may be involved in patient care delivery are illustrated in Figure 12.1.

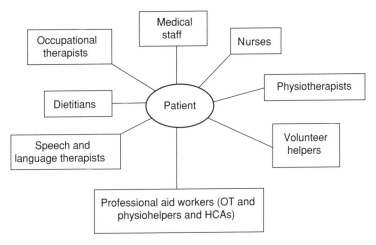

Figure 12.1   Conceptual map of team members and the patient. [Adapted from Dasgupta et al., 2005.]

The British Geriatric Society (BGS) (2006, p. 2) recommends that day hospitals should provide:

- A comprehensive assessment of frail older people
- Crisis intervention and subacute assessment with the possibility of preventing hospital admission or promoting early discharge
- Integrated assessments of health and care needs, for example, associated with decisions regarding institutional care placement or chronic disease management programmes in the community
- Treatment and rehabilitation, in particular for complex multi-faceted problems as part of community-based rehabilitation and intermediate care
- Specialist medical and nursing procedures
- A venue for speciality clinics particularly where multidisciplinary assessment is required. Examples they give such as falls clinics, movement disorder clinics, leg ulcer clinics, diabetic clinics, memory clinics, continence services and transient ischaemic episode clinics
- Rapid access admission-avoidance clinics
- Health education for the third age

Additionally, the BGS recommends that older people attending day hospitals have:

- Immediate access to senior medical opinion at all times
- Trained nursing staff with a nursing leader present in the day hospital at all times
- Immediate access to social service provision
- Immediate access to general hospital investigations such as radiology and pathology
- Daily support from allied health professional services, particularly physiotherapy and occupational therapy

- Access to other professionals such as speech and language therapist, podiatry and surgical appliances

---

Checkpoint

What groups of patients do you feel would benefit from day hospital services?

Role of the nurse

A comprehensive description of the nursing input to the rehabilitation process is conspicuous by its absence from the nursing literature, yet nurses comprise the majority of staff in most day hospitals. Indeed the role of the nurse in day hospital care appears to be largely unexplored territory. In the current climate of increased financial rigour in health services it is important that each member of the multidisciplinary team is able to justify their presence in the service as a whole and in relation to their colleagues from other disciplines. It therefore seems appropriate to explore the nursing contribution to day hospital care.

Nurses are the most prevalent health professional working in the day hospital setting (Brocklehurst, 1973; Brocklehurst and Tucker, 1980, cited in Forster et al., 2006). Vetter and Smith (1989) regard this dominance of nursing as anomalous because rehabilitation and active treatment are the most frequent modes of intervention in general day hospitals, which suggests that these authors view nursing and rehabilitation as separate entities. Other authors support this view but cite little research evidence. The nursing role is not clearly described, which may indicate its ill-defined nature, in sharp contrast to the roles of other members of the multidisciplinary team, such as physiotherapists, who are concerned with mobility and any problems which might affect it. The same goes for occupational therapists and speech therapists, with both professional groups having clearly defined roles in the rehabilitation work of the day hospital.

Nursing does not appear to have claimed any distinct role or responsibilities as its own other than the vague 'care' function. The literature seems to describe nursing in terms of specific tasks. For instance, according to Brocklehurst and Tucker (1980, cited in Forster et al., 2006), nursing 'treatment' included injections, dressings, urine testing, blood pressure recordings, eye bathing and surveillance of diet. There is no encompassing area of expertise which summarises the contribution of nurses. Nursing is aligned with medicine in these discussions, with rehabilitation as a separate entity, in the realm of the therapists from which nurses are excluded (Brocklehurst and Tucker, 1980; Cousins and Hale, 1983; Zeeli and Isaacs, 1988, cited in Forster et al., 2006). However, Brocklehurst and Tucker (1980, cited in Forster et al., 2006) identified some difficulties for nurses in accepting this situation, indicating that many would prefer to be more actively involved in rehabilitation. The aspiration of these nurses is supported by Skeet (1983), who suggests that rehabilitation is the particular responsibility of nurses working with older people and that every action should be rehabilitative in intent. There is evidence to indicate that this conviction has not been accepted to any great extent by other health care professions (Waters, 1991, cited in Booth and Waters, 1995, p. 705). For instance, with specific reference to day hospitals, Denham (1992) suggests that:

> with increasing emphasis on rehabilitation it is now appropriate to question whether nurses should still be in charge of day hospitals when the nursing role is now much reduced – a physiotherapist might be a more appropriate leader' (p. 242).

This argument can be questioned on two counts: firstly on its assumption that there has been a reduction in the importance of the nursing 'care' role, and secondly that the nursing role within day hospitals does not include rehabilitation. However, Denham (1992) is not alone in making these assumptions; in general, the literature suggests that nursing does not constitute a form of therapy or that nursing is particularly rehabilitative in nature. What then is the nursing role, particularly in view of Denham's (1992) point of why should a physiotherapist not lead the multidisciplinary team to provide integrated and collaborative care? This point made, the move to more inter-professional practice and collaboration may mean, in some instances, that the nurse may not be the right person.

Although the role of nurses within the day hospital is hard to define exactly, it has included:

- Assessment by completing a comprehensive physical and psychological review of the patient and their activities of living
- Screening blood pressure, blood sugar monitoring, weight, urinalysis and wound dressings
- Divertional therapy such as art groups, music and quizzes to aid societal engagement and interaction

Divertional therapies such as doing some art and engaging in communication enhance the strengthening of cognitive and physical skills through use of thought and hand–eye coordination and are found to be particularly beneficial for individuals who have suffered a stroke. Such activities would be offered according to individual need and choice. Figure 12.2 offers a conceptual view of the nurse's role.

Communication

Medical management of patients is usually consultant led with regular multidisciplinary team meetings ensuring dissemination of information between teams so that patients attend on the basis of need, and the benefits of their therapeutic regimens can be assessed. For example, undertaking a multidisciplinary handover at the beginning of the day utilising an adaptation of the integrated care pathway documentation (a single document incorporating a section for each of health care professional) to record patient care and treatment helps to reduce duplication of patient notes. Previous to this development, each professional involved in the care of a patient would have separate documentation which led to duplication of information. The benefits of an inter-professional approach to care in this setting lies in the fact that patients can have any number of their problems, or needs, addressed in one place. Because the patients have first-hand experience of staff working

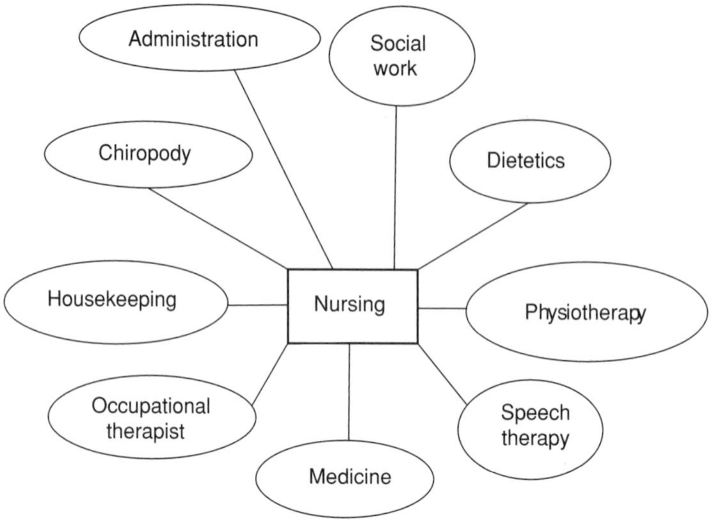

Figure 12.2   Conceptual view of the nurse's role. [Adapted from Booth, 1995.]

together who are also familiar to them, opportunities for the provision of consistent holistic care are enhanced as a therapeutic relationship develops.

Opportunity for the student

Students would have a variety of learning opportunities whilst being on a placement in this type of health care setting, including being able to observe and participate in the running of a variety of specialist outpatient clinics, rehabilitation programmes and medical interventions.

(1) Arrange to follow a patient's pathway from assessment through to treatment.
(2) Identify holistic elements of the management of the patient within the multidisciplinary environment.
(3) What strategies are important for building a therapeutic relationship in this time-limited process of care?

Health promotion

Health promotion within day hospitals is addressed within the different groups according to the individual reason for attending. For example:

Falls groups

Advice is given regarding:

- Medication.
- Diet.
- Foot care.

- Footwear.
- What to do if they did happen to fall? (This includes advice on aids and the input of other professions such as occupational therapy (OT) and physiotherapy assessments.)

(Some day hospitals have moved away from this title of the group to that of 'balance re-education group' as the patients did not like being referred to as 'fallers' (Yardley et al., 2006).)

Stroke group

Advice is provided regarding:

- Medication
- Controlling blood pressure
- Healthy diet
- Prevention of weight gain

These groups will have an inter-professional approach to the management and running of the group.

Parkinson's group

This group incorporates the Parkinson's nurse specialist to give specific, targeted advice on day-to-day management of the condition.

Respiratory group

These are continuing care groups which cater for chronic conditions. One such group may be patients with chronic obstructive airways disease (COPD) and will provide information on breathing exercises and correct inhaler technique advice, as well as general lifestyle advice.

Developments

Rapid changes in health care necessitate that these systems be flexible in order to adapt to environmental, technological and patient group evolvement without requiring continual relocating of services. In the past year day hospitals have contributed greatly towards meeting the targets for ambulatory care in line with the UK government's agenda to reduce acute bed occupancy (Black, 2006). There has been a shift in that previously excluded groups could now receive care in day hospitals, providing more intensive services for patients who do not require an inpatient admission. Examples include medical investigations, glucose-tolerance tests, infusions and drugs trials where patients require only up to an 8-hour stay and are safe to return home following treatment without an overnight stay.

In keeping with this strategic shift, day hospitals are moving away from providing services for the older person and towards day care of the adult patient. Benefits for these patients include a reduction in hospital-acquired infection and advantages associated with attendance within a day care environment (being dressed in their own clothes and being classified as ambulatory care). With this change in the role of the day hospital and the move of most rehabilitation care, previously undertaken by day hospitals, now to be delivered within community settings, day hospitals are in an ideal position to take on new roles for ambulatory care services. Therefore, a reduction in rehabilitation work and an increase in medical ambulatory care are likely to occur in the future in day hospital services.

Forster et al. (1999) highlight that:

- Patients attending day hospitals display more favourable outcomes in comparison with those receiving no comprehensive elderly care.
- Day hospitals have a generally similar impact on patient outcomes as other forms of care such as inpatient, outpatient and domiciliary services.
- Day hospital attendance may have a favourable impact on the need for long-term institutional care in comparison with other forms of care.
- A trend towards the reduced use of hospital beds is evidenced amongst the day hospital attendees in comparison with those utilizing other services/no service.
- Day hospitals appear to be more expensive than other forms of comprehensive elderly care; however, more stringent costing analyses are required to assess the extent to which these higher costs may be offset by reduced demands on hospital and institutional care resources (p. 701).

According to Black (2006) the increasing developments of community-based intermediate care teams provide an opportunity to extend the evidence-based advantages of a comprehensive assessment model in day hospitals to care for the older person in the community. In addition, this would facilitate better case findings, better medical management of step-up intermediate care patients and better coordination of care. Black (2006) also states that in the future day hospitals may become part of a hospital without walls containing day surgery, outpatient clinics, radiological and pathological investigations, advice centres, assessment rooms for therapists and integration with social services, as well as links with community matrons in the management of chronic disease. Certainly such developments would be in keeping with the current agenda of more integrated inter-professional working and the collaborative advantages that accompany this.

Out-of-hour use could be considered, in particular, in partnerships with social services, education providers and voluntary and charitable organisations. Possible uses include day centre provision, keep fit and yoga classes, stroke clubs, group meetings of organisations such as the local kidney patients association and health education groups (Black, 2006).

Adult day centres

With the changes to the role of the day hospital many services previously undertaken have been transferred and developed in day centres, including the socialisation aspect and assistance of personal hygiene. Day centres are a meeting place for all people of state retirement age, both active and frail, and managed by organisations like social services or Age Concern. A range of services and activities are available such as:

Services:

- Range of holistic services
- Hairdressing
- Assisted bathing
- Chiropody
- Hand care
- Lunch and drinks
- Hearing aid maintenance (tubing, batteries and cleaning)
- Hearing aid clinic
- Reflexology
- Library facilities
- Benefits agency, inland revenue social service advice
- Wheelchair loan
- Health authority walking aid repairs (through referrals)
- Home visits for assessment purposes
- Carers support group

Activities:

- Whist sessions
- Art classes
- Outings
- Singing for pleasure group (Silver song clubs)
- Concerts
- Bingo
- Handicraft
- Knit and natter
- Monthly dances
- Computer lessons and internet access available

Referrals for day care come from statutory and voluntary organisations, families, carers and friends in addition to requests from retired people. Some services may be subject to waiting lists and a home visit will be arranged prior to day care commencing. The centre generally recommends a 1-month trial period.

Scenario

Mr Brunt who is 70 years old is referred by his general practitioner following a recent fall (see Chapter 5 on minor injuries) to the day hospital for assessment. He arrives with his partner John who tends to talk for him. You notice that as he walks across the waiting room his gait is halting and his expression is fixed. He requires a falls assessment

(1) What are your priorities in this assessment?
(2) How would you disseminate information within the multidisciplinary team?
(3) What interventions might you consider?

Summary

Day hospitals developed rapidly in the United Kingdom in the 1960s as an important component of care provision. The model has been widely applied since in several developed countries. Day hospitals provide multidisciplinary assessment and rehabilitation in an outpatient setting and occupy a pivotal position between hospital- and community-based services. Although there is some descriptive literature on day hospital care, concern has been expressed that evidence of effectiveness is equivocal and that day hospital care can be expensive. The past few decades have seen many changes in the type of services provided. In addition to the traditional multidisciplinary rehabilitation model for the frail older person, there now exist a range of services such as specialist clinics for patients with a history of falling, Parkinson's disease, heart failure, transient ischaemic episodes, as well as rapid access clinics. Day hospitals are proving to be able to offer an effective service that moves beyond the traditional comprehensive assessment and rehabilitation of the older person to include ambulatory medical care for adult patients. Day hospitals are likely to need to respond further to the challenges of changes in health care needs and service provision in order to develop strategies that contribute to today's health care arrangements.

Acknowledgement

The author thanks Susan Holmes, Nurse Manager, Friends Day Hospital, Queen Elizabeth, The Queen Mother Hospital, Margate for advice, support and reading drafts of this chapter.

Glossary of terms

COPD
Chronic obstructive pulmonary disease is a term that refers to a group of conditions associated with chronic obstruction of airflow in the lungs. It includes bronchitis, emphysema and asthma

Glucose-tolerance test
Blood samples are drawn after an overnight fast. A glucose load is given and then specimens of blood are taken for glucose determination 1, 2 and 3 hours after glucose ingestion

Transient ischaemic episode
It is a period of cerebral dysfunction commonly manifested by a sudden loss of motor, sensory or visual function, lasting minutes up to an hour or more, but no longer than 24 hours. This is usually caused by atheromatous plaques in the carotid artery

Websites

http://www.bgs.org.uk/Publications/Compendium then select compend1-3htm
www.COPDeducation.org

http://www.dh.gov.uk/PolicyAndGuidance/HealthAndSocialCareTopics/Older
PeoplesServices/fs/en
www.headway.org.uk
www.helptheaged.org.uk
www.nos.org.uk
www.parkinsons.org.uk
www.stroke.org.uk

References

Black, D A (2006) Geriatric (Medical) Day Hospitals for Older People *Compendium Document* 4.4 [online]. Available from: http://www.bgs.org.uk/Publications/Compendium then select: compend1-3htm (accessed 15 May 2007).

Booth, J. (1995) Advantages of primary nursing in geriatric day hospitals. *British Journal of Nursing* 4(8), pp. 467–471.

Booth, J. and Waters, K. (1995) The multifaceted role of the nurse in the day hospital. *Journal Advanced Nursing* 22(4), pp. 700–706.

Brocklehurst, J.C. (1973) Role of hospital day care. *British Medical Journal* 4(886), pp. 223–225.

Dasgupta, M., Clark, N.C.T. and Bryner, C.D. (2005) Characteristics of patients who made gains at a geriatric day hospital [online]. *Archives of Gerontology and Geriatrics* 40(2), pp. 173–184. Available from: http://www.sciencedirect.com (accessed 7 February 2005).

Denham, M. (1992) Prospects for day hospitals in a changing world. *Care of the Elderly* 4(6), p. 242.

Farndale, J. (1961) *The Day Hospital Movement in Great Britain.* Oxford: Pergamon Press.

Forster, A., Young, J. and Langhorne, P. (1999) *Medical day hospital care for the elderly versus alternative forms of care.* For the Day Hospital Group. *The Cochrane Database of Systematic Reviews*, Issue 3, Art no. CD001730. DOI: 10.1002/14651858.CD001730 (accessed 15 May 2007).

Forster, A., Young, J. and Langthorne, P. (2006) *Medical day hospital care for the elderly versus alternative forms of care.* For the Day Hospital Group. The Cochrane Library. *The Cochrane Collaboration, Vol. 2. Cochrane Database of Systematic Reviews* (accessed 15 May 2007).

Department of Health (DH) (2001) *National Service Framework for Older People.* London: HMSO.

Department of Health (DH) (2003) *How Can We Help Older People Not Fall Again? Implementing the NSF Fall Standard. Support for Commissioning Good Services.* London: HMSO.

Department of Health (DH) (2004) *Better Health in Old Age: Resource Document from Professor Ian Phelp, National Director for older people's health to Secretary of State for Health.* London: HMSO.

Hershkovitz, A., Gottlieb, D., Beloosesky, Y. and Brill, S. (1 July 2003) Programme evaluation of a geriatric rehabilitation day hospital. *Clinical Rehabilitation* 17(7), pp. 750 755.

Luekenotte, A. (2000) *Gerontologic Nursing,* 2 ed. St Louis, MO: Mosby.

Potter, P.A. and Perry, A.G. (2001) *Fundamentals of Nursing,* 5 ed. St Louis, MO: Mosby.

Skeet, M. (1983) *Protecting the Health of the Elderly.* Copenhagen: World Health Organization.

The British Geriatric Society (BGS) (2006) *Geriatric (Medical) Day Hospitals for Older People BGS Compendium Document* 4.4 [online]. Available from: http://www.bgs. org.uk/Publications/Publication%20Downloads/Compen_4-4%20Day%20Hospitals.doc (accessed 14 November 2007).

Yardley, I., Donovan-Hall, M., Francis, K. and Todd, C. (2006) Older people's views of advice about falls prevention: a qualitative study. *Health Education Research* 21(4), pp. 508–517.

Chapter 13

Conclusion

Peter Ellis and Lioba Howatson-Jones

The context of the book

Throughout this book the reader has been encouraged to seek new opportunities for learning. These opportunities have included seeking information from other textbooks, journal articles, policy documents, fellow nurses and other professional colleagues as well as to reflect on new ways of working. The reader has also been encouraged to engage in meaningful dialogue with patients in order to try to gain some insight not only into the processes of care provision but also into the experience of care.

The philosophy of the book has been that the provision of care and how it is experienced is made up of a complex series of interactions which include information giving as well as being receptive to, and indeed seeking out, new sources of information and new experiences. Working within health care provision is a dynamic state of being where the practitioner, even once qualified, is permanently learning and evolving new ways of practicing, interacting and sharing knowledge.

This chapter seeks to present a simple model for these processes which places the need for criticality and reflection at the heart of practice. It further seeks to establish that the acquisition, reflection on and synthesis of knowledge is a valuable state of being for both the novice and the expert practitioner. Engagement with life-long learning, continuing personal and professional development, awareness of one's personal and professional identity, inter-professional working and a patient focus are regarded as central tenets of good-quality and continuously improving patient care.

Critical practice

Critical practice is a term familiar to all nurses. At its heart lies a willingness to engage with many sources of information using these in order to make sense of the complexities of health care provision. In this context critical should not be thought of as a state of negative thought, or fault finding, neither is it something which applies only to high-risk life-threatening situations. Criticality should be regarded as a state whereby the practitioner consciously looks for explicit links between new and old situations, between new and established knowledge. It is about joined-up thinking leading to joined-up action.

Brechin (2000, p. 25) makes the observation that:

> the challenge is to find an approach which: acknowledges the inadequacies as well as the difficulties of much current practice; recognises the major policy changes that have been taking place; welcomes the increasingly proactive role of service-users; but still values the positive motivation to provide support for others, which takes many practitioners into health and social care work in the first place.

Brechin's approach to achieving this is to develop a questioning and reflective attitude to practice which values others as equals. Fundamental to this model is the ability to build worthwhile relationships with others. Chapter 2 explored some of the communication skills required of a good health care professional. This model takes these skills to another level where open, honest communication is part of the professional relationship not only with patients, but also with colleagues, other professionals and other health and social care agencies.

The model further suggests adopting what Brechin (2000, p. 33) calls 'a not knowing approach'. Such an approach accepts that health care professionals operate in a constantly evolving field of practice and as such have to remain open to developing, or increasing, their knowledge base and engaging in learning opportunities whenever and wherever they arise. The model necessitates that health and social care professionals acknowledge that the people who they work with, both patients and colleagues, are all different. It accepts that whilst the professional may have experience of achieving high-quality outputs from care, that the experience of care and its outcomes, depend not only on what is achieved in relation to the patients conditions, but also on how they experienced that care. This healthy questioning approach to care serves to help develop personal and professional relationships as well as one's personal knowledge base.

Dialogue with other professionals, both from within the immediate team and from other agencies, is regarded as conferring a collaborative advantage (Kanter, 1994 cited in Hudson et al., 2003, p. 233). This collaborative advantage helps the professional achieve care provision which is more holistic and overcomes some of the difficulties of providing care in complex and increasingly technology-driven care settings. It might also be regarded as a positive response to some of the criticisms of poor inter-professional and agency working raised in high-profile reports such as that of Laming in to the tragic death of Victoria Climbié (Lord Laming, 2003). Developing positive working relationships which are advantageous to patient care also benefit the professionals by reducing replication of effort. They also create opportunities for learning and positive environments of care which are exciting places to work.

The advantages of good-quality dialogue with the patient include a more positive patient, and staff, experience; the ability to gain useful information from the patient pertinent to the provision of care; a greater ability to understand the patient perspective and hence engage in meaningful information giving, empowerment, advocacy and gaining of consent. The adoption of a not knowing or healthy questioning approach demonstrates to the patient that they are seen as equal partners in their care. Such partnerships are healthy and may go some way to helping overcome the barriers to trust and dialogue that have been built up around traditional interpretations of professional identity (Foster and Wilding, 2003).

Brechin (2000) regards forging relationships as the first pillar of critical practice and empowering people as the second. The nature, usefulness and philosophy behind empowerment have been explored to some extent in Chapter 2 where a practical view of empowerment was presented which sees it as part of a choices continuum with advocacy. In this model, both advocacy and empowerment recognise that the patient is the centre point of force regarding their own care. Critical engagement is about being alert and open to possibilities whilst also recognising the contribution of personal assumptions and values.

Brechin suggests that the third pillar of critical practice is 'making a difference' (2000, p. 41). As a predominantly practical professional this pillar holds great attraction for nurses. It is this pillar, however, that also creates the most challenges for the practicing professional. It is at the point of action that the nurse is presented with many challenges. What action should be taken? Why? How? And how does one decide? As well as presenting challenges, this is where a model of critical practice is at its most useful. The critical practitioner recognises that there are a number of influences on decision making in clinical practice (see Box 13.1). Furthermore, they recognise that the importance of each of these influences changes from situation to situation. They also recognise that the exercise of critical decision making is underpinned by ethical and moral principles and that they must be able to justify their decisions. That is to say they have to exercise accountability.

Morally active practice

The morally active practitioner will recognise that there are situations when some of these influences take precedence over others and that some ethical principles, like equity, always need to be applied. The ethical framework which emerges from the famous ethics textbook by Beauchamp and Childress (2001) presents a useful set of principles which the critical practitioner may decide to engage with. These principles are:

Autonomy
Justice
Beneficence
Non-maleficence

Box 13.1 Influences on decision making

Experience
   Personal and professional
      Of colleagues
      Of other professional
      Of the patient
Evidence
   From research
   From experience
Policy
   Local
   National
   Value and ethics
   Personal
   Professional
Management
   Local initiatives
   Recognising the local culture and context
Ability
   Recognising what can realistically be done
   Using available expertise
Cost
   Is it reasonable
Patient preference
   Is this well informed
   Is this reasonable
Local practice
   How things are normally done
   What resources are available

The caveat is that there is scope within these principles to assign greater or lesser importance to any one principle within any given situation. The morally active, critical practitioner should also recognise that as well as adopting such principles as central tenets of their practice they need to be aware of the potential consequences of their actions.

The diverse nature of the influences on decision making is challenging for the less experienced practitioner. Experience, practice and engagement with education, reflection and discussion with other professionals all enable the critical practitioner to not only make sense of the complexities of decision making, but relish the richness that this complexity brings to their working life.

Reflexive practice

Reflection is part of the process of developing a repertoire of decision-making skills, which lies at the core of learning criticality. Reflection may be undertaken at different levels, but research shows that it often remains at the level of practical problem solving, rather than extending into critical enquiry (Glaze, 2002). Critical reflection, in contrast, is a process of intense and deep contemplation of situations which encompasses personal contributions and that of others, within a holistic framework of practical and psychological influences and considerations. Undermann Boggs (2003, p. 56) regards critical reflection as thinking about 'one's own thinking process' in order to become aware of ways of knowing and how knowledge is used. To become reflexive is to be able to respond to situations spontaneously from a knowledgeable position that also recognises the diverse opportunities for learning.

The critical practitioner will therefore be prepared for new and challenging situations because they have explored the limits of their understanding, they have mentally rehearsed for new challenges, but they remain critically active assessing all the sources of evidence within a given situation.

For the novice practitioner, access to experienced clinical supervision can help to foster the reflective abilities and depth of insight necessary to support such a knowledgeable and critically responsive stage of the lifelong learning continuum. Such facilitation, which reviews practice with a more experienced practitioner, helps to challenge existing ways of knowing and helping the novice practitioner to consider many sources of evidence and possible actions. As health care becomes an increasingly complex endeavour extending across traditional boundaries, health professionals need to be able to look at situations more creatively and develop diverse ways of translating a variety of knowledge into their practice.

Final conclusions

This book has sought to provide the student and the trained nurse with opportunities for developing their knowledge and understanding of the care of the patient in outpatient settings. The approach of the book has been to develop something more sustainable for the reader. That is to develop an approach to practice that encourages the reader to purposefully structure that way in which they have accumulated knowledge both from practice and through more established routes of learning. This book should not be read in isolation; it has sought to reinforce, develop and lay the foundations for continuing development in the arena of understanding about the provision of care in the outpatient and day service setting. The reader has been encouraged to reflect on their own understandings, to seek out new experiences and synthesise the ideas contained within the book into what they already know.

This book has presented a philosophy of care provision which places the patient at the heart of what happens in the outpatient department and day care setting. It has shown that communication is an important part of the therapeutic relationship. It has established that the ethical practitioner will empower their patients and seek consent for the procedures that they undertake. Individual chapters have examined the changes in policy and governmental focus that have made the provision of care in the outpatient and day care setting an increasingly important and vital part of care provision in the UK. Each chapter has explored some of the specifics of care within individual arenas as well as the developed and developing roles of the nurse in the provision of care in these areas.

Individual chapters have encouraged the reader to take a broader look at the issues raised and where they fit into the bigger picture of outpatient and day care provision. The reader has also been encouraged to seek out new opportunities for learning whilst reflecting on how this new knowledge fits in with what they have already learnt.

References

Beauchamp, T.L. and Childress, J.F. (2001) *Principles of Biomedical Ethics*, 5th ed. Oxford: Oxford University Press.

Brechin, A. (2000) Introducing critical practice, in Brechin, A., Brown, H. and Eby, A. (eds) *Critical Practice in Health and Social Care*. London: Sage Publications, pp. 25–47.

Foster, P. and Wilding, P. (2003) Whither welfare professionalism?, in Reynolds, J., Henderson, J., Seden, J., Charlesworth, J. and Bullman, A. (eds) *The Managing Care Reader: A Reader*. London: Routledge, pp. 204–212.

Glaze, J.E. (2002) Stages in coming to terms with reflection: student advanced nurse practitioners' perceptions of their reflective journeys. *Journal of Advanced Nursing* 37(3), pp. 263–272.

Hudson, B., Hardy, B., Henwood, M. and Wistow, G. (2003) In pursuit of inter-agency collaboration in the public sector: what is the contribution of theory and research?, in Reynolds, J., Henderson, J., Seden, J., Charlesworth, J. and Bullman, A. (eds) *The Managing Care Reader: A Reader*. London: Routledge, pp. 232–241.

Lord Laming (2003) *The Victoria Climbie Inquiry*. London: Her Majesty's Stationary Office.

Undermann Boggs, K. (2003) Clinical judgement: applying critical thinking and ethical decision-making, in Arnold, E. and Undermann Boggs, K. (eds) *Interpersonal Relationships: Professional Communication Skills for Nurses*. St Louis: Missouri: Saunders, pp. 47–71.

Index

Note: *f* and *t* after page numbers refer to illustrations/figures or tables